Targeting Autism

WHAT WE KNOW, DON'T KNOW, AND CAN DO TO HELP YOUNG CHILDREN WITH AUTISM SPECTRUM DISORDERS

Third Edition

SHIRLEY COHEN

UNIVERSITY OF CALIFORNIA PRESS
Berkeley   Los Angeles   London

"Diagnostic Criteria for Autistic Disorder" (Appendix A) reprinted with permission from the *Diagnostic and Statistical Manual of Mental Disorders,* 4th ed., Text Revision (Washington, D.C.: American Psychiatric Association, 2000).

"Diagnostic Criteria for Asperger's Disorder" (Appendix B) reprinted with permission from the *Diagnostic and Statistical Manual of Mental Disorders,* 4th ed., Text Revision (Washington, D.C.: American Psychiatric Association, 2000).

University of California Press, one of the most distinguished university presses in the United States, enriches lives around the world by advancing scholarship in the humanities, social sciences, and natural sciences. Its activities are supported by the UC Press Foundation and by philanthropic contributions from individuals and institutions. For more information, visit www.ucpress.edu.

University of California Press
Berkeley and Los Angeles, California

University of California Press, Ltd.
London, England

© 2006 by Shirley Cohen

Library of Congress Cataloging-in-Publication Data

Cohen, Shirley, 1937–.
    Targeting autism : what we know, don't know, and can do to help young children with autism spectrum disorders / Shirley Cohen.— 3rd ed.
        p.   cm.
    Includes bibliographical references and index.
    ISBN-13 978-0-520-24838-0 (pbk. : alk. paper)
    ISBN-10 0-520-24838-4 (pbk. : alk. paper)
    1. Autism in children.   I. Title.
RJ506.A9C63   2007
618.92'85882—dc22   2006001985

Manufactured in the United States of America
16   15   14   13   12   11   10   09   08   07
10   9   8   7   6   5   4   3   2

This book is printed on New Leaf EcoBook 50, a 100% recycled fiber of which 50% is de-inked post-consumer waste, processed chlorine-free. EcoBook 50 is acid-free and meets the minimum requirements of ANSI/ASTM D5634–01 (*Permanence of Paper*).

Targeting Autism

Contents

To the real Nellie and Sean,
wherever they may be

Acknowledgments

I wish to thank parents and other family members who shared their stories with me; the adults with autism who shared their experiences through presentations, written accounts, and personal encounters; the children with autism who were my teachers; the professionals who allowed me to observe their intervention programs and answered my questions; and the friends who supported my efforts to write this book.

Prologue to the Third Edition

Targeting Autism presents a comprehensive first excursion into the world of autism. The original edition of this book was written in 1996 and early 1997. An updated edition was published in 2002. Although much has remained the same, significant developments have taken place since then. A few of the changes have had immediate impact upon the lives of young children with autism and their families. Other events had no direct effect immediately but are nonetheless exciting because of their potential for improving lives in the future. This third edition of *Targeting Autism* adds the flavor and dynamics of the autism world in the first years of the twenty-first century as well as specific information about new developments and new ways of thinking that have modified the map of autism or may do so in the near future. The puzzle of autism has still not been solved, but the elements of the puzzle are being identified and slowly assembled.

Preface to the First Edition

In late 1993 I received a telephone call at my college office from the mother of a two-year-old boy recently diagnosed as autistic. She was looking for students to work with her son in an in-home behavioral treatment program. I promised to post a notice on the "Jobs" bulletin board of the Department of Special Education. Two more mothers called me for the same purpose a short time after that, and the department chairperson also received a couple of such calls. I asked the mothers with whom I spoke what had made them choose this type of intervention and whether they had looked into other types of approaches or programs. They referred me, sometimes angrily, to a book written by Catherine Maurice, the mother of two autistic children who had "recovered" through an in-home behavioral program designed by O. Ivar Lovaas, a professor at the University of California, Los Angeles. The Lovaas treatment model was not new. Not only had I read his 1981 manual for this approach (*Teaching Developmentally Disabled Children: The ME Book*) about ten years earlier, but I had been dismayed by aspects of his approach. Yet something appeared to be happening that I wanted to understand. I read Catherine Maurice's book and—more than thirty years after my intensive involvement with autistic children—was drawn back into the world of autism.

Two autistic children I fervently wanted to help, but couldn't, haunt my memory. I was a young teacher filled with energy, a sense of mission, and faith in my own competence; and I felt particularly drawn to children who needed special attention and assistance. In 1959 I fell in love with a group of six- and seven-year-olds at a treatment and research center for children who were at that time categorized as having childhood schizophrenia or childhood psychosis. Today, almost all those children would be labeled autistic. Some of the children at this center were helped considerably and went on to enter mainstream education classes; others showed moderate improvement and went on to special education classes in public schools; a few showed very little improvement and were placed in residential treatment centers for adolescents or in institutions. The two students who have haunted my memory these many years were children I didn't help enough. Could there now really be a way to help children like Nellie and Sean?* I decided to find out.

The father of an adolescent with autism joked to his audience of parents and professionals at a conference on autism: We parents know why we're here; we had no choice. But sometimes we wonder about you professionals. The special education teacher sitting next to me answered for both of us: Autistic children get into your system and stay there.

This book is the story of autism as I put it together from the vantage point of over thirty years of professional focus on the education of young children with disabilities, including an intensive reimmersion into the study of autism in recent years. This book is not an exhaustive reference or a detailed manual. It is to serve as a sort of road map of the world of autism for parents, educators, other clinical personnel, and students. For families this book attempts to offer a broader framework and a richer context of

---

*I changed the names of individuals with autism and some details about them, unless the published literature identified them.

experiences than do the biographical case studies written by parents of autistic children. For professionals and students this book attempts to convey the challenge and fascination of autism, while also presenting the best current data and thinking on the subject.

Many stories punctuate the book. Narrative approaches have renewed stature in teaching and learning as a way of clarifying issues, putting behavior into the human context, and enriching communication about behavior. Parents, individuals with autism, and professionals use narrative to share with others what they have experienced and learned. While a single narrative may have restricted value, multiple narratives on the same subject, including biographies, case studies, and story fragments, point to important themes in defining problems and understanding dynamics.

The mysterious code of autism remains unbroken, but we now have tools that may loosen its bonds and enable many individuals with autism to emerge into a common life space with the people significant to them. We are also coming much closer to deciphering the code that turns the lives of some children into chaos and spreads havoc and despair throughout their families. This book highlights what we know, what we don't know, what we can do, what controversies exist, and what promising leads may help us achieve the goals of understanding autism and eliminating its devastating effects on the development of children.

PART ONE

What Is Autism?

1 Meeting Autism

There she moved, every day, among us but not of us, acquiescent
when we approached, untouched when we retreated, serene, detached. . . .
Existing among us, she had her being elsewhere.

(Park 1982, 12)

I visit the home of parents I recently met. Their five-year-old son is standing on his head on the couch. I go up to him, turn my head to the side, and say, "Hello, Kenneth." "Hello, Kenneth," he echoes.

I enter a room at a hotel where an informal meeting is in progress. As soon as I step through the doorway, a handsome, nicely dressed young man of perhaps seventeen walks up to me and tells me his name. The following exchange then takes place:

"What is your name?"

"Shirley."

"What is your sister's name?"

"Which sister?"

"How many sisters do you have?"

"Two."

"What are their names?"

"Paula and Sandy."

"What is your brother's name?"

"How do you know I have a brother?"

After faltering for a second, he continues, "You don't have a brother?" His attention then immediately shifts to the person who entered the room after me, and the same questioning routine begins again.

I am at a national conference on autism. Walter, a man perhaps in his mid-twenties, draws my attention. He claps loudly when anyone is introduced, and as he does so his mouth opens, his head moves from side to side, and his eyes appear to focus at a point near the ceiling. Walter and his mother are sitting only a few feet from the bluegrass band that is to play at the conference reception. As soon as the loud and lively music starts, Walter's hands begin to twist rapidly in arcs before him, the right one clockwise, the left counterclockwise. He keeps clasping his hands together, whether to stop their movement or to clap I don't know, but his hands keep breaking loose. His head turns faster and faster, keeping time with both his hands and the music. When the music ends, Walter's movements slow to a stop. He looks at the ceiling briefly and then sits quietly.

A woman who has a PhD is making a presentation: Temple Grandin has written two books about herself as well as numerous articles on autism. She is also the subject of an intensive case study in the book *An Anthropologist on Mars* (1995) by the neurologist Oliver Sacks. Temple Grandin is a person with autism.

We glimpse here a few of the many faces of autism. One of the most striking aspects of the condition (or conditions) referred to as "autism" is its variability. What then do people identified as having autism have in common? What does the term mean if it encompasses such heterogeneity? What is the concept behind the label? To answer this question we need to look across several perspectives—those of researchers, clinicians, parents, and adults with autism.

We can begin by studying the "bible" of diagnostic categories and labels, the latest version of the American Psychiatric Association's *Diagnostic and Statistical Manual of Mental Disorders*, DSM-IV-TR, published in 2000. DSM-IV-TR doesn't refer to autism; rather, it refers to *pervasive developmental disorders,* which include five categories: autistic disorder, Asperger's disorder, pervasive developmental disorder not otherwise specified, childhood disintegrative disorder, and Rett's disorder. The term "pervasive developmental disorders" is meant to indicate "severe and pervasive impairment in several areas of development: reciprocal social interaction skills, communication skills, or the presence of stereo-typed behavior, interests, and activities" (American Psychiatric Association 2000, 69). In practice, the term "autism spectrum disorders" has largely replaced the term "pervasive developmental disorders," except in those instances when the very low-incidence conditions of Rett's disorder or childhood disintegrative disorder are the focus.

Let's look at what *autistic disorder* may mean through examples provided by parents.

Qualitative impairment in social interaction. Catherine Maurice describes the social isolation of her infant daughter:

> Anne-Marie was not shy: she was largely oblivious to people, and would sometimes actually avoid them, including, a lot of the time, her own mother. She drifted toward solitary spaces: the corners of a room, behind the curtains, behind the armchair. If I was somewhere else in the apart-ment, she never sought me out. . . .
> Worst of all, perhaps, was the lack of that primary connection: the sweet steady gazing into one's eyes that we began to see all around us in other toddlers. . . . Sometimes I would catch her gazing in my direc-tion and would start up, eager to respond to her invitation, to meet her look. But her eyes, frighteningly, were focused upon some middle dis-tance, somewhere between me and the wall behind me. She wasn't see-ing me at all. She was looking right through me! (Maurice 1993, 31, 33)

Qualitative impairments in communication. Clara Park describes her daugh-ter's language at age two and then at age twenty-three. At two, her daughter Jessy used words, but infrequently and not to communicate. "She had no idea of language as a tool that could cause things to happen" (1982, 74). As she reached twenty-three, Jessy's communication problems were still striking:

Anybody who hears Jessy speak more than a word or two realizes that something is wrong. She has learned English as a foreign tongue, though far more slowly, and she still speaks it as a stranger. The more excited she is about what she has to say, the more her speech deteriorates; her attention cannot stretch to cover both what she is saying and how she is saying it. Pronouns get scrambled: "you" for "I," "she" for "he," "they" for "we." Articles and tenses are confused or disappear, verbs lose their inflections or are omitted altogether. (Park 1982, 292)

Restricted repetitive and stereotyped patterns of behavior, interests, and activities. "We watched him as he rocked his body and spun every round object he could find," recalls Barry Kaufman, describing his not yet two-year-old son's repetitive behavior (1976, 62). Judy Barron writes of her infant son:

He was drawn to odd things. He'd crawl past a brightly colored selection of toys to get to the furnace register. Once there he would stick his fingers into the slots and watch his fingers move. There was a hole in the wooden floor of his bedroom that riveted his attention. He'd put his finger into that and wiggle it around for hours. (Barron and Barron 1992, 13)

Six-year-old Paul McDonnell became obsessed with light bulbs, his mother, Jane, tells us:

His light bulb collection had grown to include not only incandescent household light bulbs, but also fluorescent bulbs, black lights, infrared and ultraviolet bulbs, and flashcubes: three hundred seventy-two in all. He kept many of his light bulbs in a basket by his bed, and every night he tried out different bulbs. (McDonnell 1993, 154)

As an adolescent Temple Grandin became fixated on squeeze chutes for cattle, an obsession that she later transformed into a therapeutic device to calm herself and others.

All autistic children do not act exactly like the children described here. Not all are as cut off from people as Anne-Marie Maurice was; not all have to struggle as hard as Jessy Park did to use language for communication; and the stereotyped interests of children with autism vary widely.

See appendix A for the specific combinations of behavioral indicators that professionals use to arrive at a diagnosis of autistic disorder.

High-functioning autism by another name is one way of thinking about *Asperger's disorder*, but DSM-IV-TR treats Asperger's disorder as a separate category of pervasive developmental disorders distinct in some ways from autistic disorder. Although the two conditions share some core characteristics—namely, severe impairment in social interaction and restricted repetitive patterns of behavior, interests, and activities—Asperger's disorder, unlike autistic disorder, is not marked by severe delays in language acquisition or cognitive development during the child's first three years. When the child with Asperger's disorder begins preschool or approaches school age, problems with social communication often become quite apparent. The label "Asperger's disorder," more commonly referred to as "Asperger syndrome," has come into wide use in the United States only since the mid to late 1990s. Prior to that, children and adolescents who today are identified as having Asperger syndrome would likely have been diagnosed as having emotional disturbance, behavior disorder, and/or attention-deficit/hyperactivity disorder. Other labels used in the past to classify those children and adolescents were schizoid personality and nonverbal learning disabilities.

Individuals with Asperger syndrome are often "loners." Although most show interest in making friends after the early childhood years, their attempts to do so are frequently unsuccessful. Contributing to such failures are insensitivity to other people's feelings and nonverbal communications, as well as long-winded, one-sided "conversations" about their own favorite interests. In spite of good academic performance in most areas, or even giftedness, children with Asperger syndrome are commonly viewed as odd, and they often lack even a rudimentary sense of what is socially appropriate. Kenneth Hall, who at age ten produced a book about himself (*Asperger Syndrome, the Universe and Everything*), writes: "If I am unhappy about something I tell the truth. Like if I am fed up with a visitor. Or if I dislike something. Or if I dislike a person. Or if someone does or says something stupid. . . . Sometimes adults get annoyed when I am honest" (2001, 66).

Individuals with Asperger syndrome also often appear to lack common sense, as in Rita's case. Rita was not identified as needing special education services when she was a child; academically she functioned at grade level in elementary school. But in adolescence her behavior became increasingly age-inappropriate or eccentric, and she was referred for evaluation. Rita tried hard to copy the dress and chatter of her classmates, but she couldn't keep up with the rapid pace of their communications and couldn't master the process of achieving the "right" look. Her first attempts to use makeup produced exaggerated and grotesque results. At age eighteen, Rita moved to a group home where the staff focused on developing skills for independent living and work. On one of her weekend trips to her family home, Rita seemed to be trying to apply some of the skills she had been taught. She entered a fish store and, after a substantial period of consideration, indicated to the proprietor the particular fish she wanted. After the fish had been weighed and she had been given the price, Rita stated that she was now going home to ask her mother if she could buy it.

Young children who do not strictly meet the criteria for autistic disorder or any other pervasive developmental disability are often assigned the label "PDD," which is a shorthand version of the term *"pervasive developmental disorder not otherwise specified"* (PDD-NOS). This label indicates that the child displays impairment in reciprocal social interaction and in one of the two other defining areas for pervasive developmental disorders without fitting the picture of another pervasive developmental disorder. By age six or seven, many children with this label have been reclassified as having either autistic disorder or Asperger syndrome.

Sometimes well-meaning professionals use the term "PDD" or "PDD-NOS" with very young children when they feel that a diagnosis of autistic disorder or autism would be premature, and they want to protect families from the frightening associations commonly linked to these terms. PDD is presented as a serious, multifaceted problem in development, but one that is not quite as severe as autism. At times, the concern that leads to the use of the PDD label can have unintended negative effects, such as leaving parents confused or making it more difficult to obtain intensive early intervention services for the child. Another reason for use of the PDD label is parents' growing awareness of the importance of early identification of developmental disabilities and the availability of intervention services for very young children with disabilities. While it is possible to identify many children with pervasive developmental disorders at eighteen to twenty-four months of age or even younger, at such an age the distinction between the various categories within autism spectrum disorders is not always clear.

Most people, when they have heard anything at all about autism, have a particular image of it that represents only one of the faces of autism. While the full range of variations in autism may not be apparent in early childhood, one difference can be clearly seen: some children with autism appear different almost from birth, while others appear to develop normally for a period of time and then begin to regress. By the time her daughter was one month old, Annabel Stehli (author of *Sound of a Miracle*) was sure that something was wrong. Time only added confirmation. Georgie did not grasp her mother's finger or look at her or smile or snuggle against her when she was being held. Judy Barron (author of *There's a Boy in Here*) reported a similar experience with her son Sean, who never seemed to want to be held, squirming, twisting, and pushing against her as if he felt trapped when she picked him up.

Some professionals who are considered experts on autism have in the past stated that what seems to be late-onset regressive-type autism may in fact reflect delay in detection owing to parental denial or lack of sophistication. That may sometimes be the case. I think back to what the mother of my student Nellie said to me over thirty years ago. Nellie was doing all right until she went to nursery school, her mother told me, implying that something had happened at nursery school to cause her daughter's autistic behavior. Yet home films viewed by the clinical staff had shown a two-year-old Nellie, before any nursery school experience, hiding behind furniture and people, not looking or smiling at anyone, not playing with anyone. Nellie's mother was trying to account for an unexplainable loss that caused great grief. However, recent studies of the early development of children with autism that have analyzed videotapes taken between eight and twelve months of age demonstrate that many parents were right: about 25 percent of these children appeared to be developing typically until sometime during their second year (Werner and Dawson 2005). It was the professionals who doubted parental reports who were proven wrong about late-onset autism.

There's no question of delayed detection creating a false appearance of late onset in Jordan Schulze's case. His early development was too advanced and its reversal too sharp a contrast. His parents' sense of loss was excruciatingly exacerbated by development suddenly halted and then reversed.

> A clear-eyed boy of nineteen months is pointing to the gaily decorated tree in my living room. "Christmas lights, Daddy," he says as he reaches up to touch the bulbs. "This one is green. This one is blue." Jordan goes through all the colors, carefully pointing out the names of each that he touches. From across the room my wife, Jill, beams as she listens to these first words of the season from our first child. . . .
>
> The here-and-now version of the happy toddler is the seven-year-old boy who, on this day alone, has bitten the school bus driver, flung himself on the floor in a fit of rage in the grocery store, spent nearly half an hour tapping toys on his teeth, and occupied himself in his last waking hour flushing the toilet over twenty times. (Schulze 1993, i–ii)

Childhood disintegrative disorder, or *Heller's syndrome,* is a rare pervasive developmental disorder, and it has a very poor prognosis. According to DSM-IV-TR its essential feature is "a marked regression in multiple areas of functioning following a period of at least two years of apparently normal development." The areas affected include language, social skills or adaptive behavior, play, motor skills, and bowel or bladder control; and this condition is "usually associated with severe mental retardation" (American Psychiatric Association 2000, 77, 78). There are no known biological markers that can be used to differentiate childhood disintegrative disorder from autistic disorder.

Craig Schulze is an educator with a PhD in human development whose son was diagnosed as autistic, but who came to believe that his son had childhood disintegrative disorder. In his 1993 book Schulze describes the deterioration of his young son and his own fruitless struggle to return Jordan to his first life: "It is as if he has died from one existence and returned in another form. . . . Psychologists, neurologists, self-styled gurus, teachers (American and Japanese), relatives and friends, even our own intuitions had joined in a continuing chorus of 'We Shall Overcome.' Now the harmony is gone, and the tune is flat, and the voices are silent" (42, 147).

"He" is the common personal pronoun in books on autism, but that usage does not reflect gender bias. Autism is largely a male disorder, approximately four times more prevalent among boys than among girls. But that is not the case for the last category of pervasive developmental disorders. *Rett's disorder,* or *Rett syndrome,* the fifth pervasive developmental disorder presented in DSM-IV-TR, shares several features with both autistic disorder of late onset and childhood disintegrative disorder, but it is virtually exclusive to females. Rett syndrome is a progressive, genetically based neurological disorder in which infants who seemed to be developing typically begin to lose ground sometime after five months of age, with resultant severe impairments in language, cognition, hand usage, and gross motor functioning. An X-linked gene whose mutations lead to Rett syndrome has been identified.

Why are there differences in time of onset and the course of development in autism spectrum disorders? The answer to this question is still elusive. But one of the factors that seems to account for some differences in the course of development is the presence or absence of mental retardation. Some children with autism function as if they have mental retardation, even with intensive early intervention, while others show clear signs of good cognitive ability in multiple areas. However, it is often difficult to determine the cognitive ability of a young child with autism. Aside from the broader issues about the conceptualization of intelligence and the meaning of IQ, how are we to assess intelligence in children who may have no functional speech or any other organized communicative system, who rarely look at people or attend to verbal directions or imitate movements?

Occasionally a child will show unusual abilities that seem to provide clues. Some young autistic children are *hyperlexic*—that is, they learn to read at an early age without formal teaching, in spite of a general delay in language development, although this reading may be largely word naming with little comprehension. Other children may show different kinds of evidence of prodigious rote memory. Astounding abilities in art, music, and calendar calculations have been noted in autistic individuals who otherwise appear to be moderately to severely mentally retarded; and "islets" of competence in such areas as mathematics are not uncommon in autistic individuals who otherwise function at a level considered to indicate mild mental retardation. (Sometimes early signs of autism are not recognized because of such islets of competence in the young child.)

IQ in young children does seem to matter. A performance IQ approaching 70, combined with some functional language by age five, seems to be associated with a greater likelihood that the child will have a better developmental outcome. But autistic children are idiosyncratic; they break all rules. Some autistic children are nonverbal until well beyond age five and are considered to be mentally retarded, and then they begin to communicate and prove everyone wrong. Yet the variability of intelligence among individuals with autism is unquestionable. Many young children with autism make slow and limited progress in learning even with intensive intervention, while others have gone from treatment programs to challenging educational programs and on to college studies in such areas as mathematics or science.

IS AUTISM BECOMING MORE COMMON?

"There are, due to a tragic accident of nature, children with autism who live in society, but who for some as yet ill-understood reasons cannot profit much from the social stimulation provided by loving and caring parents" (Volkmar 1993, 40). Who are these children? How many are there?

In 2005 the Centers for Disease Control and Prevention of the U.S. Department of Health and Human Services estimated that up to 500,000 individuals between birth and age twenty-one had an autism spectrum disorder, although many of the younger children in this population had not yet been diagnosed and classified. This estimate was arrived at by using a rate of occurrence of 1 in 166 or about 60–62 per 10,000, which was the rate found in several recent studies that considered the entire autism spectrum. This rate is dramatically higher than those found in earlier studies. For years, the generally accepted rate of occurrence was 4–5 per 10,000, although individual studies sometimes reported higher figures; by the mid to late 1990s, the widely accepted rate was 10–15 per 10,000. While large increases in prevalence have been reported for autistic disorder, the greatest increase in prevalence has occurred in the milder forms of autism spectrum disorders (Chakrabarti and Fombonne 2001).

Autism used to be considered a low-incidence disorder. Now it is referred to as one of the most common childhood conditions within the category of serious developmental disorders, surpassing such conditions as cerebral palsy and Down syndrome. Clearly, something real has been happening to bring about such a large rise in the reported prevalence of autism spectrum disorders. The question still to be resolved is how much of this rise represents a true increase in prevalence and how much reflects other factors such as earlier identification, greater willingness by physicians and psychologists to use diagnostic labels on the autistic spectrum with young children, and modifications in diagnostic categories and criteria. The large increase in Asperger syndrome, in particular, may at least to some extent reflect more familiarity with this diagnostic label and better identification.

One mother raised a question about classification and labeling within the autism spectrum that cannot be answered until the condition we now call autism is better understood. She questions whether high-functioning individuals with autism should be grouped with individuals who have severe autistic disorder and whose behavior and functioning are quite different (Gilbert 1995, 4). The issue here is whether these are distinct conditions or different intensities of the same disorder. Do they have the same etiology, or are the underlying factors different? The answers to these questions are still unknown.

ETIOLOGY: THE SEARCH CONTINUES

The etiology of autism is still not well understood, but autism appears to have a strong and complex genetic foundation. It is more common in some families than in most others. Studies have shown that the prevalence of autism among siblings of autistic individuals is about 6 percent, substantially higher than in the general population; and the concordance rate for autism in identical twins is much higher than in nonidentical twins. There is no difference in prevalence rate between nonidentical twins and other siblings; but if one identical twin has autism, it is very likely that the other has an autism spectrum disorder as well. This may be the case as much as 90 percent of the time. A higher than expected frequency of Asperger syndrome has been found in the families of high-functioning individuals with autism, and Oliver Sacks refers to an entire family of individuals on the autism spectrum—the gifted parents and older son with Asperger syndrome, the younger son with classic autism—who, "between the serious business of life," flapped their arms, jumped on a trampoline, and screamed (1995, 244). Moreover, parents or other close relatives with mild versions of autism have been identified in a good number of families of children with autism; and even when no other person in a family has an autism spectrum disorder, the family may have a higher than expected prevalence of individuals with social and communicative impairments. These findings strengthen the hypothesis that autism has a genetic base.

If autism spectrum disorders are, in fact, more common today than they were in earlier decades, what is causing this increase? The answer presented most frequently during the past few years by parents is vaccines. Why vaccines? The hypothesized genetic basis of autism did not seem to adequately account for the increase in prevalence reported in the past few years. What many parents began to notice was a close connection in time between the administration of a triple live-virus vaccine for measles, mumps, and rubella (MMR) when their children were twelve to fifteen months old and a deterioration in their babies' functioning. The medical community explained this association as a noncausal coincidence in time, but Andrew Wakefield, an English doctor, hypothesized that the MMR vaccine might be triggering regressive autism in genetically vulnerable children.

Vaccines had long been recognized as causing problems in a tiny fraction of young children, and the Centers for Disease Control and Prevention and the U.S. Food and Drug Administration maintain a Vaccine Adverse Event Reporting System. Before the MMR vaccine became the focus of controversy in regard to autism, the pertussis toxin in the diphtheria-tetanus-pertussis (DTP) vaccine was identified as posing a risk of brain damage for a very tiny percentage of young children, and action was taken to modify the pertussis formulation in the version of this vaccine that is now in use (DTaP). However, the number of children harmed by vaccines was considered so low relative to the imposing benefits of vaccination that this problem of adverse reactions received only limited attention from the medical community.

Parents and their supporters have raised multiple questions about vaccines. While the role of the MMR vaccine as a possible trigger for autism was being examined and debated, another possible trigger associated with vaccines was identified. This time the target of parental concern was the inclusion of thimerosal, a substance containing a form of mercury, as a preservative in some of the vaccines administered to children during their first and second years. Although a review conducted by the Food and Drug Administration concluded that no harm had taken place because of vaccines containing thimerosal, the agency nonetheless recommended that, as a precautionary measure, the use of thimerosal should be reduced or eliminated. In 1999 an agreement was forged with vaccine manufacturers to accomplish that goal. As of 2005, only one childhood vaccine, the flu vaccine, still contained thimerosal, and a thimerosal-free version of this vaccine had become available.

While most children who received vaccines containing thimerosal had no long-term adverse outcomes, many parents whose autistic children had been given such vaccines believed that the mercury in thimerosal had overwhelmed their children's immune systems and led to autism. These parents argued that the total amount of mercury to which their babies had been exposed through vaccines far exceeded safety standards. Researchers pointed out that the standards parents referred to were for a different type of mercury—methylmercury rather than the ethylmercury in thimerosal—and that methylmercury crosses the blood-brain barrier more easily. Moreover, research studies of the MMR vaccine (which did not contain thimerosal) and of vaccines containing thimerosal appeared not to support the parents' belief that such vaccines were triggering autism. The 2004 final report of the Immunization Safety Review Committee of the Institute of Medicine, which was commissioned to review all evidence on vaccines and autism, concluded that the available epidemiological evidence did not support the hypothesis of a causal relationship between vaccines and autism.

In 2005 the book *Evidence of Harm* was published. Written by a science and health reporter, David Kirby, this book and its title became a rallying point for anguished and angry parents who believed that the medical establishment, which was supposed to protect their children, had instead greatly diminished their children's lives. Each research report that rejected the thimerosal hypothesis was itself subjected to a point-by-point critical review by parent groups such as Safe Minds. Parents were not about to give up.

If thimerosal-containing vaccines triggered autism in genetically susceptible children, the incidence of autism spectrum disorders in young children should have begun decreasing in 2005, when children who had received much less of this substance through vaccines reached four or so years of age. As of 2005 there were conflicting reports about whether this was occurring. The picture should become much clearer by 2007, when most children in the United States who received very little thimerosal through vaccines will be six years of age or older.

While the Institute of Medicine and other prestigious medical groups have not accepted the hypothesis that there is a causal relationship between vaccines and autism in genetically vulnerable children, professionals should not stop listening to parents. It was a parent, K. H. Schulte-Hillen, who pushed doctors to consider the drug thalidomide as the possible cause of a sudden rash of infants born with deformed or missing limbs in the early 1960s in West Germany (1969). Had it not been for this father of one such infant, many more children would have been born with such congenital deformities. Heredity was also an explanation given by some doctors for this condition prior to Schulte-Hillen's search for a cause. We do not yet understand the mechanism underlying late-onset autism, and vaccines may or may not be a significant part of that picture, but parents are excellent sources of information and hypotheses that should be thoroughly examined. There are multiple possible environmental triggers for autism, both prenatal and postnatal. In fact, there is some research evidence to support the idea that thalidomide, taken at a specific period during early pregnancy, might be a prenatal trigger for autism. About one-third of the "thalidomide babies" born in the early 1960s had not only physical deformities but autistic characteristics as well.

Perhaps the most encouraging development in the search for the causes of autism spectrum disorders is the significant expansion of funding for research in this area in recent years. These dollars are coming from the National Institutes of Health (NIH), from states such as California, from large private donations, and from the fund-raising activities of parent-led organizations dedicated to the mission of identifying the causes of autism. Studies that may help us clarify the role of genetic, prenatal, and postnatal factors in the etiology of autism spectrum disorders are being carried out today at numerous sites across the country.

ARE AUTISM SPECTRUM DISORDERS DISTINCT FROM ALL OTHER DEVELOPMENTAL DISORDERS?

Questions can be raised about the differential diagnosis of autism and other disabilities outside the spectrum of pervasive developmental disorders that may mimic the appearance of autism. Labels indicating categories of disability are most useful when all individuals identified by a particular label exhibit the defining characteristics of that category, when there are clear boundaries between categories, and when an individual who fits into one such category will not meet the criteria for another one. Unfortunately, autism eludes this framework. Autism should be viewed as a working label. When more is known about the cause or causes of this disorder, the label "autism" may be replaced by several labels, or the way in which we think about this syndrome and related developmental disabilities may be dramatically altered.

Landau-Kleffner syndrome is a disorder that mimics late-onset regressive autism in some ways. The outstanding feature of this syndrome is loss of language after a period of normal development, usually of more than two years and sometimes as long as seven years. On March 9, 1995, an ABC news program called *Day One* included a segment on Landau-Kleffner syndrome. For weeks after it aired, Thomas Jefferson University Hospital in Philadelphia was overwhelmed with telephone calls from parents for Gerry Stefanatos, director of the Center for Clinical and Developmental Neurophysiology, who had been featured in the television program. What had mobilized these parents was a rekindling of hope for the children lost to autism of late onset, children who had been developing as normally expected until perhaps eighteen or twenty months of age, when their development seemed to change course. Babies stopped using the words they had already acquired, stopped acquiring new words, stopped trying to communicate through smiles or gestures that they wanted to be picked up or played with, stopped snuggling up to their mothers to receive hugs and kisses, and stopped offering any of their own.

What parents heard and saw on the *Day One* program that gave them hope was a boy who had been labeled "autistic," but who had apparently regained his developmental momentum after being rediagnosed with Landau-Kleffner syndrome and treated for this condition. At around age two, T. J. Voeltz had "stopped talking and began to disappear" into his own world. His mother was told that there was nothing medicine could do for her son, who had incurable brain damage; she needed to get on with her life. But Kathy Voeltz did not heed these words, and eventually, at a conference on autism, she heard a speaker say that anyone who knew a child who used to talk should look into Landau-Kleffner syndrome. She did. After testing, her son's diagnosis was changed, and he was treated with the drug ACTH.

Two years later, eight-year-old T. J. Voeltz was in a second grade class. He spoke; he played; he learned. He could do most of the things that a boy his age is expected to do. His parents believe that several months of treatment had given T. J. a second chance at a normal life. It is what thousands of parents of autistic children have dreamed of. To parents, the saving grace of Landau-Kleffner syndrome is that medication can sometimes reverse its downward course, whereas no medication has been identified as effective in reversing the core features of autism. A basic question can be raised about the boundary between autism and Landau-Kleffner syndrome: are these totally distinct conditions, or can their boundaries touch or even overlap?

Landau-Kleffner syndrome, also sometimes referred to as *acquired epileptic aphasia,* is a condition of very low incidence. Epilepsy is present most of the time, and abnormalities in brain wave patterns are central to the diagnosis of this condition. What complicates the differential diagnosis of late-onset autism and Landau-Kleffner syndrome is the fact that children with autism also have higher than normal rates of abnormal electroencephalograms (EEGs) and epilepsy. Seizure disorders have been identified in at least 25 percent of individuals with autism by early adulthood, with two peak periods of incidence, one in early childhood and one in adolescence (Volkmar and Wiesner 2004); and some types of seizures are not recognized by families or intervention personnel. Instead, these seizures are mistaken for symptoms of autism such as poor attention, abnormal eye gaze, and stereotyped behavior. Furthermore, many children diagnosed with autism have not had EEGs; and even those who have had an EEG may not have had a twenty-four-hour (sleep) EEG, which is often essential for detection of abnormal brain waves in young children. A twenty-four-hour EEG should be part of an evaluation whenever a child presents with autism of late onset that is not responsive to intensive intervention.

Landau-Kleffner syndrome may be treated with anticonvulsants or corticosteroids such as prednisone. The reported outcomes for children treated with these medications range from complete, dramatic remission of symptoms to partial recovery with mild language disorder to continued severe speech/language impairment. Major improvements in language are rare, and some medical professionals considered to be autism experts advise against using anticonvulsant medications and corticosteroids unless the child has epilepsy, since these medications may have significant negative side effects. However, in a November 2005 presentation at a conference on autism, the well-regarded neurologist Michael Chez reported that his treatment of young autistic children who had abnormal brain waves with low dosages of the anticonvulsant Depakote may have prevented seizure disorders from developing in these children during adolescence.

A father who has guided the care of his severely disabled son for over thirty years said to me, "Yes, my son has autism, but that's just one of his problems." To understand what that father meant we have to consider the concept of comorbidity—co-occurring conditions or behavioral symptoms that occur together at greater than chance levels. Several conditions are comorbid with autism, and the continuing issue in autism is whether these conditions reflect a common underlying cause or whether one condition leads to the other. About 10 percent of children with autism have a known genetic disorder such as fragile X syndrome or tuberous sclerosis.

Fragile X syndrome is a disorder defined by a particular genetic marker, namely a fragile site on the X chromosome. This syndrome is associated with mental retardation in males and with social and communicative dysfunctions characteristic of autism. The prevalence of fragile X syndrome in males who meet the criteria for autism is about 6 percent; and at least 15 percent of children with fragile X syndrome meet the criteria for autism. Walter, the young man whose behavior at a conference reception caught my attention, has fragile X syndrome, a fact that his mother learned only after he was given the simple screening test for this condition that has been available since the early 1990s. As a child, Walter was diagnosed with autism, but no other condition was identified. Today Walter is considered a man with fragile X syndrome and autism. Little in his life changed because of this modification in his diagnosis after he reached adulthood. He continued to work in a supported employment program operated by an autism agency, and his relationship to his family remained the same. What did change was the addition of a new concern: Walter's mother worried that her daughter might be a carrier of fragile X syndrome and could transmit this genetic disorder to any children she might have.

Tuberous sclerosis is a rare genetic disorder involving unusual tissue growth and variable other symptoms that may include seizures and developmental delays. Approximately one-third of children with tuberous sclerosis meet the criteria for autism, although a very small percentage of children with autism spectrum disorders have tuberous sclerosis.

Obsessive-compulsive disorder is another condition that shares some distinctive features with autism. The compulsive repetitive behaviors of individuals with obsessive-compulsive disorder sometimes cannot be distinguished from the rituals and repetitive fixed routines often found in children and adults with autism. Jeffrey's father describes his four-year-old son's behavior:

> I went to father's night at my Jeffrey's pre-school. He was playing with a Fisher-Price toy, a schoolhouse, but his play was strange. He stood before the toy, jumped up and down, and flapped his arms as if excited by it. . . . When the jumping stopped, he would put his arms together and wiggle his fingers just above eye level. . . . He did this for 35 minutes. (Rapoport 1989, 29–30)

The description of Jeffrey's stereotyped behavior makes it easy to begin thinking of autism, but Jeffrey did not have the severe difficulties in communication that are characteristic of autism. In this way he was more like a child with Asperger syndrome, but that label didn't fit either because Jeffrey did not have a deficit in reciprocal social interaction. He was not only affectionate toward his parents, as some young autistic children are, he also tried to act in ways that pleased them, and he recognized the unusual nature of his compulsions. "Mommy, why do I play with strings?" asked this child who would dangle strings in front of his eyes for four hours a day (31). Jeffrey was diagnosed as having obsessive-compulsive disorder, and his stereotyped behavior was controlled with medication. Some individuals with autism meet the criteria for obsessive-compulsive disorder as well.

Attention-deficit/hyperactivity disorder (ADHD) is a condition that appears to be comorbid with some types of autism spectrum disorders. Diane Kennedy, the mother of three sons diagnosed with ADHD, understood this label in regard to her two older sons, but it didn't seem adequate to describe the more complex functioning of her youngest son. Yes, he was impulsive, hyperactive, and inattentive, but at age three he also did not have direct eye contact, was extremely sensitive to sensory stimuli, had numerous temper tantrums, bit other children without apparent provocation, and insisted on sameness. In her book *The ADHD-Autism Connection*, Kennedy describes her mission as increasing "awareness about the similarities between ADHD and autistic spectrum disorders, especially Asperger syndrome," so as to "facilitate more productive dialogue, more accurate diagnoses, and more effective treatment" (2002, 2). More recently, some researchers have pointed to cases in which autistic disorder and PDD-NOS in young children evolve into ADHD in middle childhood after intensive treatment aimed at the core characteristics of autism. These researchers propose various hypotheses that may account for this change, including the idea that a PDD-ADHD subtype exists, with attention difficulties becoming more salient after social and language problems are ameliorated (Fein et al. 2005).

Other conditions may also be comorbid with autism, *Tourette's disorder* among them. The motor tics that are a central feature of Tourette's disorder may be mistaken for the stereotyped behaviors in autism.

Comorbid conditions are not found in all individuals with autism, but they do occur at higher rates than in the general population. From a parent's point of view such comorbidity implies the likelihood of more difficulties and perhaps a less optimistic developmental outlook. For the researcher, comorbidity is a clue in the search for the causes of autism.

And so, after examining conditions difficult to differentiate from autism, associated with autism, and overlapping with autism, we come back to two basic questions: what is autism, and what causes autism? Autism is a name, a label we assign to a set of observed behaviors. Those behaviors may reflect multiple origins and may affect the neurological system and other body systems to different degrees. Our current conceptualization of autism, the way we define and categorize it, may change as we learn more about its origins and the pathways between those origins and the observed behavior to which we currently attach that label.

As Marie Bristol, a speaker from NIH, said at a 1996 conference when she addressed the question of what causes autism: "The short answer is that we don't know." But, she added, we have some good hunches. That is still the situation today. We know that autism does *not* come from something bad that parents did to their children, as was generally believed in the 1950s and 1960s, but it may come from parents in a different way. One of the strong beliefs among researchers today is that autism, or a susceptibility to autism, is inherited and may be triggered by a variety of environmental factors, prenatal or postnatal. Autism also appears to reflect a combination of differences in both structural and functional aspects of the nervous system. Researchers are hard at work trying to identify these differences and trace the path that led to them. We do not yet know the cause or causes of autism, but answers to critical issues surrounding its origins are beginning to emerge.

2 Having Autism

In 1950 I was labeled autistic and groped my way
from the far side of darkness.

(Grandin and Scariano 1986, 15)

A highly articulate cum laude graduate of one of the most prestigious universities, who was diagnosed as autistic in childhood, had been speaking to his audience for about twenty minutes. "I grew up on the fringes of typical society," he told us. "I always thought I was weird and strange. . . . Many of us wind up on the fringes of society. Even those of us with college degrees are unemployed or underemployed. . . .

"We, whose labels were dropped, are just becoming aware of ourselves," he continued. "There aren't many of us. . . . Some of us have discovered e-mail. We don't have to deal with the anxiety-provoking aspects of conversation—the other person stops and it's your turn. . . . We joke about '1,499 out of every 1,500 people being born with typicality.' . . . When it comes to forming relationships with 'typicals,'" he related, "it doesn't often happen. . . . People sense that something is different."

Individuals with autism are a highly studied population. They are observed and tested, treated and tested; their parents are questioned; their blood is examined, and increasingly so too are their neurological systems, thanks to newer brain-imaging techniques. There are probably thousands of articles on the subject of what goes on inside the minds and bodies of autistic people, and yet the answers are incomplete. We can describe the range of behavioral characteristics of individuals with autism and delineate ways in which their behavior is different, strange, even deficient. We formulate hypotheses to account for these differences and test these hypotheses. Sometimes we even listen to adults with autism as they try to tell us how they have experienced their own autism.

Individuals with autism describing their experiences? It sounds like a contradiction. Individuals with autism have difficulties in communication, in relating to others; they have little insight or ability to understand others' viewpoints. Are they even aware of how they differ? Autistic people whose ability to communicate is very limited or absent may not help us answer that question, but those individuals who are considered higher-functioning are aware of these differences, as several have told us in their autobiographical accounts.

Multiple books and numerous articles and presentations make Temple Grandin the superstar of autistic communicators. In her late fifties now, she has come a long way, understanding her differentness and developing strategies to cope with the expectations of the outside world. Donna Williams, with books, articles, interviews, and a web site, is Temple's closest rival. Other biographical accounts are more modest—Paul McDonnell's coda to his mother's account of his life (McDonnell 1993); the comments of Sean Barron interwoven with those of his mother in their jointly authored book (Barron and Barron 1992); and parts of articles or chapters by others. Asperger syndrome has drawn more attention in recent years, with books by individuals as young as ten (Hall 2001) and by adults with doctorates, such as Liane Holliday Willey (1999) and Stephen Shore (2003).

We are cautioned not to rely too much on the content of accounts by people with autism; it may mislead us. We should consider possible limitations in the autistic person's insight and the applicability of the experiences of this tiny subgroup of highly able autistic individuals (Happe 1991). Yes, it's a skewed sample that does not represent a large segment of the population of autistic individuals. Yet we can learn from it. The perspective of these "insiders" may shed light not only on their own experiences but also on those of somewhat less able autistic individuals. Their accounts, used in tandem with the findings of professionals and the perceptions of parents, illuminate the experience of being autistic.

To illustrate the tandem use of insider and outsider perspectives, let's look at the thinking of highly able individuals with autism or Asperger syndrome. Temple Grandin, in her book *Thinking in Pictures*, reports: "Language and words are alien ways of thinking for me. All my thoughts are like playing different tapes in the videocassette recorder in my imagination. Before I researched other people's thinking methods, I assumed that everybody thought in pictures" (1995, 142). Research data and clinical observations support the idea that visual ideation is common among individuals with autism, and many educational programs for young autistic children incorporate visual teaching and learning strategies to capitalize on it. A study of introspection in three adults with Asperger syndrome found that all three described their inner experiences exclusively in visual images, whereas the normal subjects studied earlier had reported multiple types of inner experiences, including verbal thinking. One autistic subject referred to images as the shapes of his thoughts (Hurlburt, Happe, and Frith 1994). Reports by individuals with autism and research by professionals can be used together productively to provide insight into the dynamics of autism.

Certain themes jump out of the biographical accounts of people with autism spectrum disorders. They are reiterated by almost every individual. Fear, confusion, pain, and the arduousness of life permeate the descriptions of childhood. Kenneth Hall, a gifted ten-year-old with Asperger syndrome, writes: "Sometimes I can get a lot of depression. These times make me feel that life is a downward spiral. Every bit of my body feels grey shafts of lightning pain and I feel like banging my head on the wall or something" (2001, 100). An autistic man looking back at his childhood remembers: "Fear was my biggest problem. It was a terrible feeling" (Donovan 1971, 101). When Jerry, a thirty-one-year-old man who had been diagnosed as autistic at age four by Leo Kanner, is interviewed about his memories of childhood, he recalls confusion and terror (Bemporad 1979). A twenty-two-year-old man diagnosed as autistic at age two states: "I was afraid of everything!" (Volkmar and Cohen 1985, 49). Donna Williams reports that "the more I became aware of the world around me, the more I became afraid" (1992, 5). Sean Barron shares this recollection: "Sometimes I sit and reflect on my life so far. I remember the fear that was always with me, the confusion, the chaos, and the storminess of my life with my family" (Barron and Barron 1992, 257). An eighteen-year-old woman writes: "In the beginning, when I was a child, life was very difficult" (DePaolo 1995, 9). A forty-one-year-old man with Asperger syndrome reports: "I fear that people are not going to be pleased with me. I fear that if I do the wrong thing or say the wrong thing I will undo all the progress I have made so far" (Dewey 1991, 202).

Part of the fear in childhood came from the apparent instability of the world. Everything appeared to be always changing. "Nothing seemed constant; everything was unpredictable and strange," according to Jerry (Bemporad 1979, 192). Paul McDonnell recalls: "When my mom moved the furniture in the house I got very, very upset. I hated the change. I felt like I was not at home any more" (1993, 348). Another adult with autism asserts: "I hate change. I always have, I always will" (McKean 1994, 45).

Rituals are developed to ensure stability and predictability. Everything has to be in a certain place. Events have to occur in a certain order. People have to act in specified ways. Control becomes critical to ensuring predictability and stability. Liane Willey explains:

> As long as things followed a set of rules, I could play along. Rules were—and are—great friends of mine. . . . You know where you stand with rules and you know how to act with rules. Trouble is, rules change and if they do not, people break them. . . . When they are broken, the whole world turns upside down. (Willey 1999, 43)

By setting out exacting prescriptions for behavior, some individuals with autism have made their homes hellish for other family members.

Certainty is a goal, but certainty is often evasive. Repetition offers the key to certainty. Paul McDonnell states:

> In the past I used to ask the same question over and over and I used to drive my parents crazy by doing that! I wanted to hear the same answer over and over because I was never sure of anything. . . . I wanted an exact answer to everything; uncertainty used to drive me crazy. (McDonnell 1993, 327)

"I loved repetition," Sean Barron relates. "Every time I turned on a light I knew what would happen. When I flipped the switch, the light went on. It gave me a wonderful feeling of security because it was exactly the same each time" (Barron and Barron 1992, 20).

People are not like light switches. They don't act exactly the same each time. Their behavior cannot be easily understood or predicted by autistic individuals, particularly not by autistic children. This may be part of the reason why people may have little meaning for many young children with autism.

> People bothered me. I didn't know what they were for or what they would do to me. They were not always the same and I had no security with them at all. Even a person who was always nice to me might be different sometimes. Things didn't fit together to me with people. Even when I saw them a lot, they were still in pieces, and I couldn't connect them to anything.
>
> Thinking back, I believe that when I was a child, up to the age of five or six, I would not have been able to pick out my mother from a group of other women. I never really looked at her. (Barron and Barron 1992, 20–21)

Negative feelings toward people sometimes developed because people intruded into the special world of the autistic child and interrupted the child's pleasurable and comforting activities. "I hated my mother becaus [sic] she try [sic] to stop me from being in my world and doing what I liked," a young man writes (Volkmar and Cohen 1985, 49). "I remember my mother telling me not to do things I loved," Sean Barron tells us. His parents were always "interrupting me and interfering with me" (Barron and Barron 1992, 21). Donna Williams relates, "I felt secure in 'my world' and hated anything that tried to call me out of there. . . . People, no matter how good, had no chance to compete" (1994b, 8).

What are the experiences that engross and comfort and give pleasure to young children with autism? Donna Williams describes her childhood world as the "pleasant, beautiful, and hypnotic experiences of mere color, sensation, and sound" (1992, 129). Temple Grandin offers the following description:

> I could sit on the beach for hours dribbling sand through my fingers. . . . Each particle of sand intrigued me. . . . Other times I scrutinized each line in my finger, following one as if it were a road map.
> I enjoyed twirling myself around or spinning coins or lids round and round and round. Intensely preoccupied with the movement of the spinning coin or lid, I saw nothing. . . . People around me were transparent. And no sound intruded on my fixation. (Grandin and Scariano 1986, 22)

Not understanding words or their purpose contributes greatly to the confusion of young children with autism and hinders the development of connectedness to other people. Donna Williams explains this:

> Words were no problem, but other people's expectations for me to respond to them were. This would have required my understanding what was said. . . . "What do you think you're doing?" came the voice. Knowing I must respond in order to get rid of this annoyance, I would compromise, repeating "What do you think you're doing?" addressed to no one in particular. "Don't repeat everything I say," scolded the voice. Sensing a need to respond, I'd reply: "Don't repeat everything I say." (Williams 1992, 4)

Bill Donovan, a "near-normal" adult with autism reports, "I learned to talk at 4. I didn't learn to communicate until 11 or 12" (1971, 102). What he meant by this statement was that he, like Donna Williams, parroted words without understanding their meaning or purpose. Not being able to talk was the hardest part of his childhood, he relates. "I destroyed things . . . *because I couldn't talk*" (100).

Understanding the speech of others did not guarantee that a child could produce speech. Steffie DePaolo writes: "I am an autistic person and for a long time, I was completely unable to express myself . . . the only solution I had was anger. Then came the tantrums" (1995, 9). "As an autistic child, difficulty in speaking was one of my greatest problems," Temple Grandin relates. "Although I could understand everything people said, my responses were limited. I'd try, but most of the time no spoken words came. . . . My mother and teachers wondered why I screamed. Screaming was the only way I could communicate" (Grandin and Scariano 1986, 18, 106). Perhaps the worst aspect of not being able to speak, bright autistic children found, was being unable to show how much they knew and understood.

Jim Sinclair, a leader in the self-advocacy movement of persons with autism spectrum disorders, describes his inability to use speech to communicate until he was twelve: "I simply didn't know . . . what talking was for. . . . Speech therapy was just a lot of meaningless drills in repeating meaningless sounds for incomprehensible reasons. I had no idea that this could be a way to exchange meaning with other minds" (1992, 296). Speech, which we think of as an innate ability of human beings, appears to be no more natural to these autistic children than it is for children born deaf.

"Feeling different" is an almost universal experience among those adults who report to us on their feelings. A young man with Asperger syndrome told one audience that he grew up thinking he had a curse on him. Paul McDonnell writes: "I always knew I was different from other kids, I just didn't know what that difference was. For years I guessed I was retarded, mildly retarded. . . . That's what kids always called me" (1993, 327). "I have believed for so long that I was abnormal, retarded, inferior," Sean Barron writes (1992, 232). Feelings of "rage, shame, and hatred" toward oneself sometimes accompany this perception (Bovee 1995, 6). Ten-year-old Kenneth Hall tells us: "I always knew I was different and that I wasn't quite like other children. It's hard to say exactly how I knew. . . . Other children seemed to behave differently, play differently and talk differently, but I didn't know why" (2001, 14).

Many individuals with autism who try to explain the ways in which they are different refer to their sensations, to the way they experience sensory input. The common denominator appears to be unusual sensitivity to sensory stimuli and susceptibility to sensory overload—sounds are unbearably loud and sometimes frightening, odors may be overpowering, touch may be painful, sunlight disabling, and combinations of sensory input overwhelming.

The narrative of Darren White begins as follows: "This autobiography consists of information about my hearing and eyesight playing tricks on me." He then describes these tricks:

> I was rarely able to hear sentences because my hearing distorted them. I was sometimes able to hear a word or two at the start and understand it and then the next lot of words sort of merged into one another and I could not make head or tail of it. . . . Sometimes when other kids spoke to me I could scarcely hear them and sometimes they sounded like bullets. . . .
>
> It was a very bright day and very hot. My eyesight blurred several times that day and once I could see no more than a yard in front. . . . I broke my collarbone falling off a radiator. My eyes were showing a wide windowsill where the radiator was and I sat down falling off instantly. (White and White 1987, 224–25)

Liane Willey reports that as a young child she often found it impossible even to touch some objects, and she was assaulted by noise and light:

> I hated stiff things, satiny things, scratchy things. . . . I routinely stripped off everything I had on even if we were in a public place. I constantly threw my shoes away. . . . I ripped the tags right out of my clothing even though I knew I would get in trouble. . . .
>
> I also found many noises and bright lights nearly impossible to bear. High frequencies and brassy, tin sounds clawed my nerves. . . . Bright lights, mid-day sun, reflected lights, strobe lights, flickering lights, fluorescent lights; each seemed to sear my eyes. . . . My head would feel tight, my stomach would churn, and my pulse would run my heart ragged until I found a safety zone. (Willey 1999, 25–26)

A thirteen-year-old boy reports the approach of trains five to ten minutes before they pass his home, long before his parents can hear their approach. This same boy in describing touch reports: "It hurts . . . it's too much" (Cesaroni and Garber 1991, 306). A mother of an autistic child who herself has characteristics of autism states:

> I have cringed so many times when people came at me for a hug. I
> taught myself to tolerate this because people always seem to do it. . . .
> When I am touched unexpectedly or when I do not want to be, I can
> easily go into overload. This is comparable to having one's chalkboard
> completely erased and being left to stare at a blank board. At school,
> if I was touched while I was being taught, my brain immediately shut
> down. (Donnelly 1994, 7)

Kenneth Hall describes his early school experience: "I just hated the classroom. The noise annoyed me. At the time the sound of the children's chatter was like dynamite going off in my ears" (2001, 39). In a presentation at an autism conference, Jean-Paul Bovee, who has two master's degrees, told the audience that he could actively participate in a great conversation. He could also maintain eye contact. What he could not do was to engage in both of these acts simultaneously. "You need to choose which one you want," he told his audience (Adams 2005, 273). In a 2005 presentation at a symposium in New York City, Temple Grandin told her audience that a normal environment (for some individuals on the spectrum) is like living near a jackhammer. Donna Williams was still frequently overwhelmed by sensory stimulation in adulthood. She relates one such example:

> I had just come from another classroom where I had been tortured by
> sharp white fluorescent light, which made reflections bounce off every-
> thing. It made the room race busily in a constant state of change. Light
> and shadow dancing on people's faces as they spoke turned the scene
> into an animated cartoon. Now, in this noisy classroom, I felt I was
> standing at the meeting point of several long tunnels. Blah-blah-blah
> echoed, bouncing noise wall to wall. I looked at the cheerful, placid
> faces of the others; clearly I was the freak. (Williams 1994b, 76)

Susan Bryson, a researcher, commented on such hypersensitivity. She suggests that the perceptual world has an unusually strong pull in autism. "It is as if sensory information is too salient," and this may induce a state of overarousal that obstructs the mind and distorts information uptake (2005, 35). Another adaptation to the overwhelming salience of sensations is to periodically retreat. A sixteen-year-old with Asperger syndrome explains this behavior in a poem.

My Corner
Samuel Abram, 1999

You have taken me out of my corner
And I do not like it.
You say my corner is a problem to me,
My corner is a need.
A need to save me from the rest of the room.
A room without thought.
Whereas there is plenty of thought in my corner.
My corner is where I can be renewed.
Renewed to go into the room.
But the room can be tiresome
As I yearn for that corner.
The corner of thought and renewal.
Maybe later I will go into the room
As everybody else did,
But for now,
Leave me alone in my corner.

Unusual sensitivity to sensory stimuli is, however, only one of the problems individuals with autism describe. Autism is a pervasive disorder affecting all systems of functioning, Donna Williams reminds us (1994a). To Jim Sinclair the crux of the difference between individuals with autism and others lies in what others know without being taught:

> Simple, basic skills such as recognizing people and things presuppose even simpler, more basic skills such as knowing how to attach meaning to visual stimuli. Understanding speech requires knowing how to process sounds—which first requires recognizing sounds as things that can be processed, and recognizing processing as a way to extract order from chaos. Producing speech (or producing any other kind of motor behavior) requires keeping track of all the body parts involved, and coordinating all their movements. Producing any behavior in response to any perception requires monitoring and coordinating all the inputs and outputs at once, and doing it fast enough to keep up with changing inputs that may call for changing outputs. Do you have to remember to plug in your eyes in order to make sense of what you're seeing?. . . .
>
> These are the gaps that I notice most often; gaps between what is expected to be learned and what is assumed to be already understood. (Sinclair 1992, 295)

Making sense of emotions is one of these gaps. Paul McDonnell writes, "I just CAN'T understand human emotions, no matter how hard I try" (1993, 347). Donna Williams explains:

> I wanted to understand emotions. I had dictionary definitions for most of them and cartoon caricatures of others. . . . I also had trouble reading what other people felt. I could make some translations, though. If people's voices got louder, faster, or went up, they were angry. If tears rolled down their faces, or the sides of their mouths hung down, they were sad. If they were shaking, they were perhaps frightened, sick, or cold. . . .
>
> The most important thing was to check if people were angry. "Angry" had the worst and most invasive consequences. . . . "Are you angry?" I asked Dr. Marek, as his voice changed. "No Donna, I'm not angry," he replied for the fiftieth time. (Williams 1994b, 104)

People with autism appear to process faces differently than most other people do, and their face recognition and discrimination abilities are generally poor. Temple Grandin has "a terrible time recognizing people's faces" (Grandin and Johnson 2005, 107). Data from research studies seem to show that children with autism spectrum disorders process pictures of faces using feature-by-feature-based strategies for matching rather than the Gestalt approach used by typical peers. Typical peers also process faces significantly more quickly than they process abstract designs, while this distinction is minimal in children on the spectrum (Serra et al. 2003). Processing emotional expression and eye gaze appears to be particularly challenging for children on the spectrum. When Temple Grandin was younger, she could not interpret even the simplest expressions of emotion, Oliver Sacks reports from his meeting with her (1995); she learned to decode such expressions later in her life.

Expressing emotions can be a challenge too, as Stephen Shore reports:

> During my undergraduate days I underwent a few counseling sessions. . . . Several times the social worker asked me how I felt about what she was talking about because she said she could not tell by reading my face. . . .
>
> When dealing with emotionally charged issues, I often sense that there is something important to be worked out; however, I feel an over-

whelming conflict. Perhaps this is because emotions are a sort of "second" language to me. Not only do I have to decode the words on the verbal channel, I also have to deal with the nonverbal channel consisting of body language, facial expressions and tone of voice. To further confuse things, what is actually being said may be different from what is implied by vocal inflections and other components of the nonverbal channel. In other words, having to "read between the lines" confuses things.

When this happens, I know that something is going on but I'm not sure what it is. I want to do something about it, but not only am I unsure of what to do, I don't know how to do it. As a result . . . a shut-down occurs in the communication arena. I become unable to speak. (Shore 2003, 121)

Another of the gaps Jim Sinclair refers to is in making connections. Connections don't come easily to individuals with autism, and this gap affects all aspects of relating to the world. Professionals refer to difficulty with abstraction and generalization. Each event is perceived as distinct from all others. The categorizing that goes on in the minds of most of us all of the time—the automatic connecting of events and people that seem to go together—either doesn't happen or happens in different ways in individuals with autism. Temple Grandin reports that she had to construct her own personal library of these connections, event by event, in order to cope effectively. Donna Williams notes:

I would learn how to tackle a given situation in one context but be lost when confronted by the same situation in another context. Things just didn't translate. If I learned something while I was standing with a woman in a kitchen and it was summer and it was daytime, the lesson wouldn't be triggered in a similar situation if I was standing with a man in another room and it was winter and it was nighttime. (Williams 1994b, 64)

Difficulty in making connections contributes greatly to one of the core problems in autism, namely, reciprocal social interaction. Reciprocal social interaction presupposes a common set of perceptions and understandings that is often missing when autistic and nonautistic adults attempt to communicate. Jim Sinclair provides this insight:

The extent to which communication occurs in the course of my interactions seems to depend on how effectively I am able to identify discrepancies in understanding and to "translate" both my own and the other person's terms to make sure we're both focusing on the same thing at the same time. (Cesaroni and Garber 1991, 311)

Donna Williams describes her own difficulty in communicating:

I would often talk on and on about something that interested me. . . . I really was not interested in discussing anything; nor did I expect answers or opinions from the other person, and I would often ignore them or talk over them if they interrupted. . . . If I had to ask questions, it was as though I did so to the air. (Williams 1992, 51)

Temple Grandin's way of communicating entailed translating the wordless pictures that represented her thinking into stock statements that she had "on tape" inside her head. In high school her classmates referred to her as the Tape Recorder.

Those kids who called me Tape Recorder were right about me. They were mean, but they were right. I *am* a tape recorder. That's how I'm able to talk. The reason I don't sound like a tape recorder anymore is that I have so many stock phrases and sentences I can move around in new combinations. All my public speaking has been a great help. When I got criticisms saying I always gave the same speech, I started moving my slides around. That moved my phrases around, too. (Grandin and Johnson 2005, 18)

Communication difficulties and the lack of implicit knowledge of social conventions and codes make the process of connecting with other persons enormously costly in time and energy for the individual with autism. Temple Grandin reports that she had to learn these "implicit" social skills, like Data on *Star Trek:*

I am like Data, the android man, on "Star Trek, the Next Generation." As he accumulates more information, he has a greater understanding of social relationships. I am a scientist who has to learn the strange ways of an alien culture. . . . When I encounter a new social situation, I have to scan my memory and look for previous experiences that were similar. As I accumulate more memories, I become more and more skilled at predicting how other people will act in a particular situation. (Grandin 1995, 147)

It is the absence of this common set of perceptions and understandings, the implicit knowledge of social conventions and codes acquired during the course of childhood and adolescent development in most individuals, that leads individuals with autism to feel alien. Temple Grandin, who supplied the title for the Oliver Sacks book *An Anthropologist on Mars* in the course of describing her experiences, was not the first and is far from the only adult with autism to use an alien metaphor in trying to convey the autistic experience. Jim Sinclair reports:

> After reading Temple Grandin's autobiography . . . someone asked me if I thought a cattle chute would have helped me. I said I didn't need a cattle chute, I needed an orientation manual for extraterrestrials. Being autistic does not mean being inhuman. But it does mean being alien. It means that what is normal for other people is not normal for me, and what is normal for me is not normal for other people. In some ways I am terribly ill-equipped to survive in this world, like an extraterrestrial stranded without an orientation manual. (Sinclair 1992, 302)

Sean Barron tells us that at age fifteen, "I still didn't have a clue as to how people talked to one another. Not for the first time, I felt like an alien from outer space—I had no more idea how to communicate with people than a creature from another planet" (Barron and Barron 1992, 198).

In somewhat less striking language, other adults communicate similar experiences. A woman with a graduate degree reports: "I was never *quite* sure how to handle certain situations. It is very difficult for even a high-functioning autistic adult to know exactly when to say something, when to ask for help, or when to remain quiet. To such a person, life is a game in which the rules are constantly changing without rhyme or reason" (Carpenter 1992, 291). Liane Willey tells us that "human relationships usually take me beyond my limits. They wear me out. They scatter my thoughts. They make me worry about what I have just said and what they have just said, and how or if that all fits together . . . the whole thing drives me to total distraction and anxiety" (1999, 69).

Yet at some point all these individuals decided to try to "make it" in the alien world of "neurotypicals," to find some way to learn the rules and develop the necessary skills and coping mechanisms. For some, this happened at a specific point in time as a clear, conscious decision. Imitation of typical people was a major strategy to accomplish their goal.

> I was 14. I set my will (to) be normal like everybody else. (I) look(ed) up to people in school and did what they did to be accepted and put (up) more of a show to hide the problems and be Normal. . . . My interests were destroyed becouse [sic] I thought they wernt [sic] normal. (Volkmar and Cohen 1985, 51)

Sean Barron describes his attempts:

> I spent an awful lot of time wishing I were a different person. Why couldn't I be normal? More than anything I wanted to change all my behavior. . . . I started having "corrective" conversations with myself.
> I went on a crusade. . . . I declared war! I was going to fight against all the behaviors I had obeyed all my life. (Barron and Barron 1992, 161, 232)

Some autistic persons have more ambivalence about trying to be normal. In an author's note at the beginning of her book *Nobody Nowhere,* Donna Williams writes:

> This is a story of two battles, a battle to keep out of "the world" and a battle to join it. It tells of the battles within my own world and the battle lines, tactics used, and the casualties of my private war against others.
> This is my attempt at a truce, the conditions of which are on my terms. (Williams 1992)

She had learned that her survival rested on "refining the act of acting normal"; but "on the inside I knew that by definition this meant that whatever and whoever I was naturally was unworthy of acceptance, belonging, or even life" (1992, 80). In a television interview on CBS in 1994, she talked about giving up the mimicry of others that was central to her attempt to learn to live in the normal world so that she could find her own self; she was no longer willing to maintain a facade of normality.

"Being almost 'normal' is not easy," Jean-Paul Bovee tells us (1995, 6). Jim Sinclair tells us more about this in his poem:

I built a bridge
out of nowhere, across nothingness
and wondered if there would be something on the other side.
I built a bridge
out of fog, across darkness
and hoped that there would be light on the other side.
I built a bridge
out of despair, across oblivion
and knew that there would be hope on the other side.
I built a bridge out of helplessness, across chaos
and trusted that there would be strength on the other side.
I built a bridge
out of hell, across terror
and it was a good bridge, a strong bridge,
a beautiful bridge.
It was a bridge I built myself,
with only my hands for tools, my obstinacy for supports
my faith for spans, and my blood for rivets.
I built a bridge, and crossed it,
but there was no one there to meet me on the other side.

(Cesaroni and Garber 1991, 311–12)

Thomas McKean puts it another way in his poem "Build Me a Bridge": he comes from a different world; he wants to be part of this world; but he, himself, can't build the bridge needed to join that world.

I have known that you and I
have never been quite the same.
And I used to look up at the stars at night
and wonder which one was from where I came.
Because you seem to be part of another world
and I will never know what it's made of.
Unless you build me a bridge, build me a bridge,
build me a bridge out of love. . . .

(McKean 1994, 43)

While adults with autism are working on crossing bridges, they are also telling "neurotypicals" that they want to be who they are; their autism is part of their core, they say. "When do we stop trying to change

people?" asks Jean-Paul Bovee, the conference presenter with two master's degrees. "I'm perfect the way I am," he adds (Adams 2005, 277).

Talking about the adults on the spectrum she has met, Liane Willey says:

> We all have our own thoughts on just how important it is to fit in. Some
> of us have no desire to walk the NT [neurotypical] walk. Some of us are
> very intent on becoming more NT than aspie. Still others of us are happy
> to play NT and live aspie. (Willey 2002, 36)

Some young adults have found a niche for themselves within the
Asperger networks that have sprung up during the last few years. At
their retreats and when they gather at meetings, there is no need to pretend to be normal. Liane Willey, after striving so mightily to be typical for
so long, tells us:

> Aspie. I have grown rather attached to that word. I like the way it
> sounds. I like the way it rolls off my lips as if I am whispering a grand
> secret, for in some ways that is exactly what I am doing, the moment I
> sound the word aloud. Aspie tells my secret for it describes who I am . . .
> in an elastic sort of way. It does not lock me in to a norm . . . it means
> different . . . not less, not bad, not unworthy or incapable . . . just differ-
> ent. (Willey 2002, 155)

3 Life Cycles

> When our son's autism was diagnosed . . . we didn't even know if he'd
> ever learn to talk. . . . By the time he graduated from elementary school,
> he had no discernible behavioral or academic problems. But that was
> from a distance.
>
> *(LaZebnik 2005)*

What can I expect for my child's future? parents ask—or fear to ask but
are told anyway. Frequently, the forecast includes continued significant
impairment, multiple problems, separateness from nondisabled peers,
and perhaps lifelong special service needs. This picture is sometimes
what the future holds for children with autism disorder, but not always;
and such a future looms before autistic children much less often today
than it did ten or fifteen years ago. No single pattern of development and
adult outcome characterizes the autistic condition. There are many possible patterns, and many factors—some controllable, some not—shape
those patterns. Parents need to know this. So too do the physicians and
others—professionals and nonprofessionals—who interact with children who have autism and their families. This chapter addresses some of
the developmental patterns and trajectories noted in individuals with
autism spectrum disorders.

INFANTS AND TODDLERS

Until relatively recently, when the urgent need for early intervention was recognized, the diagnosis of autism was usually deferred until a child was three years old. No speech at age two? "Give your child a chance," doctors would say; "children develop at different rates." No reaching out to others? "Some children are shy; you're being overanxious." By age two and a half, they might add, "He's a little slow developmentally." But the mothers of these children often knew, or at least strongly suspected, that something was seriously wrong; and in many cases they sensed this almost from the time they brought their babies home. How did they know? What were the clues they "picked up" that others did not recognize until much later?

Differences in babies' temperaments are apparent even in their first days of life. Some infants are quite fussy, while others lie quietly, hardly moving; some cry most of the time as if in great discomfort, while others cry occasionally and with less vigor; some can be soothed easily by being picked up or fed, while others seem impervious to almost all attempts to soothe them. Researchers have studied these differences and have found them to reflect long-lasting patterns of behavior.

No single pattern of infant behavior characterizes babies who are later identified as autistic. But two patterns are commonly reported: the very easy or "perfect" baby—quiet, undemanding, apparently content with little attention from caregivers—and the very irritable baby who resists soothing and does not establish eye contact. Some of these babies don't like being held and reject all attempts at cuddling or other forms of physical contact, even arching their bodies away from their parents. Of course, many such babies grow into happy and healthy children; there is no one-to-one correspondence between these early patterns and later outcomes. Just the same, these early patterns provide a kind of first alert that a baby may need some special help with its development.

Tony was an irritable baby who was later recognized as having autistic characteristics. In her book *Fighting for Tony*, Mary Callahan describes the constant crying that marked his first two and a half years:

Each day Tony's crying spells grew longer and more frequent. . . . Most days he cried for an hour or two in the morning, about four at dinnertime and another hour during the night. . . . Our pediatrician talked of colic and immature nervous systems. He said it wouldn't last more than six weeks. On the day that Tony turned six weeks old, I took him to the doctor in the middle of what turned out to be nine straight hours of crying. (Callahan 1987, 20, 21)

Let's look at some of the other early clues that infants with autism may provide. Right from the start, something very basic about relating to people seems not to be working. Common characteristics of children under age three who are diagnosed as having autism include little or no eye contact, lack of responsiveness to voice (often leading to suspicion of deafness), and apparent obliviousness to people.

Typically developing infants are interested in human faces almost from birth. Young babies smile at and vocalize to their mothers. The normally developing infant turns toward an adult who has begun speaking and studies that person's face. After a while infants add anticipatory gestures, lifting their arms to be picked up. A pattern of reciprocal interaction develops, with mother and baby being the focus of each other's attention and regulating their behavior in response to each other. When the baby cries, the mother is soothing. When the mother is playful, the baby smiles or laughs. The parent's face becomes a source of important information for the baby in situations of uncertainty, as when a new toy is presented or an unfamiliar adult seeks close contact.

This process of social referencing, that is, getting cues from the parent or other caregiver, helps guide the infant's responses. Near the end of the first year, the infant also intentionally uses communicative signals to direct the parent's attention to interesting objects and events, to share those experiences. The infant may point to a dog passing by or hold out a toy and vocalize and then check to find out if the adult is looking at it. This joint attention, along with social referencing and reciprocal interaction, provides the foundation for later social relatedness and communication. Deficits in joint attention may be predictive of delayed language development.

Infants with autism are much less active participants in joint attention, social referencing, and reciprocal interactive behavior with their parents and other caregivers. In the case of late-onset regressive autism, such behaviors are lost or significantly reduced sometime after the first year. Studies of home videotapes of infants during first birthday parties demonstrate that infants with autism attend less to faces than typical infants do. Unlike typically developing children, young children with autism do not show different brain electrical responses to photographs of their mothers and photographs of women they don't know (Dawson et al. 2002). Such lack of attention to faces and poor early facial recognition may reflect differences in the neurological system. These babies don't effectively use eye contact, facial expressions, and gestures in relating to their parents and others. Nor does the human voice appear to carry special meaning or attract any special attention. One of the earliest signs of autism is a baby's failure to orient to voice or to respond when his or her name is called.

One theory that attempts to explain this difference postulates that the process of regulating arousal is impaired in the autistic infant. One of the staunchest supporters of this theory is Stanley Greenspan, considered by many to be the mentor of developmental intervention with very young children. Based on his work with hundreds of infants and toddlers, Greenspan developed multiple concepts that are relevant to an understanding of pervasive developmental disorders, particularly the idea of a "regulatory-sensory processing disorder" (Greenspan and Wieder 1998, 2005).

A *regulatory-sensory processing disorder* is an inability to process sensations well, that is, to take them in, modulate (adapt to) them, and comprehend them, while staying calm and attentive. Infants with such disorders may overreact or underreact to noises and bright lights; may show "tactile defensiveness," stiffening and arching their bodies to avoid the physical handling involved in being dressed or held; may underreact or overreact to pain; and often have severe difficulty with auditory processing and the processing of multisensory experiences. Greenspan believes that severe regulatory-sensory processing dysfunction interferes with communication and the formation of relationships by hindering the development of shared attention and reciprocal gesturing between a baby and his or her parents. Thus, he links the concept of a "neurodevelopmental disorder of relating and communicating" to a regulatory-sensory processing dysfunction that has derailed the infant's core capacities in these areas. With different kinds of words, Greenspan describes the early sensory experiences reported by Donna Williams, Temple Grandin, Sean Barron, Paul McDonnell, Jim Sinclair, and other persons with autism encountered in the previous chapter.

Why does this connection matter? What implications does it have? Let's consider the finding that many infants with autism appear not to recognize their parents until well beyond the age when most typically developing babies can do so, even well beyond the point when most babies with mental retardation can differentiate their parents from strangers. Greenspan's explanation might point out that, to an infant, the visual image of the human face usually appears simultaneously with auditory, tactile, and often kinesthetic stimuli; parents talk or sing to their babies while they stroke or rock them and seek to establish eye contact. Thus, the infant who can't cope with multisensory stimuli may be overwhelmed.

Greenspan's conceptualization has implications for the selection of early intervention strategies. For example, an initial strategy might be careful observation of the baby's responses to various stimuli, followed by a reduction in the types and levels of stimulation that appear to cause the infant to withdraw or become upset. Sensory stimulation that the baby seems to favor would be continued. Later, the baby would be very gradually reintroduced to the types of stimuli that were not well tolerated earlier.

Geraldine Dawson of the University of Washington also believes that a baby's ability to adapt to various types, levels, and combinations of sensory stimuli is central to healthy development (1991). Normally developing infants react to people and other stimuli with either orienting or aversive responses—turning toward and attending to the stimulus, or turning away from the person or object. An orienting response is the typical reaction to stimuli of mild intensity, such as soft speech and gentle rocking; whereas an aversive response is a common reaction to very intense stimuli, such as loud shouting. Infants with autism may, however, have abnormal arousal patterns: stimuli that arouse interest in most babies may meet an aversive response such as gaze avoidance in the autistic baby.

Is the optimal level of novelty lower for the autistic infant? Most infants are interested in stimuli that are slightly different from what they have previously experienced but not ones that are totally novel. What they seem to seek are a few familiar features. Thus, we could conceive of an optimal level of novelty along with an optimal range of stimulation. For children with autism, the optimal level of novelty may be lower. This possibility is supported both by the marked distress that autistic children show over minor changes in their environments and by their restricted range of interests. The narrow range of optimal stimulation and novelty for autistic children may also help explain their difficulty in understanding people and participating in social situations. Novelty and unpredictability are much more closely associated with social stimuli than with objects.

Infants and toddlers with autism spectrum disorders also often exhibit difficulties with motor organization, although this is not a defining characteristic. The lack of a pointing gesture, which infants typically develop before age one, and the poor motor imitation displayed by some infants and toddlers with autism are other indications of developmental problems that interfere with the achievement of age-appropriate behavior.

As the child with autism moves from infancy and toddlerhood to the preschool years, ages three to five, we see a child who lacks a solid foundation for social interaction and communication, who may well have problems in modulating stimuli, and who may have motor problems as well. Some new areas of delayed development are also likely to become apparent: the absence of age-appropriate play, and the presence of stereotyped behaviors, that is, repetitive motor sequences that have no obvious function, such as hand flapping or the lining up of object parts. These difficulties mark an inauspicious entry into the preschool years. Parents of some of these children, noting their differences in development, marshal all possible resources to obtain intensive early intervention services for their children.

The toddler who will later be diagnosed as having Asperger syndrome will likely be talking now and may even appear to be gifted because of precocious verbal language. But this child too will be showing signs of differences in development, often with limited eye-to-eye gaze and other aspects of nonverbal communication, little of the reciprocal give and take of conversation, and little interest in other children. Because parents are usually less concerned about these children before age three, few of such toddlers undergo diagnostic evaluations unless they have begun to have major tantrums or "meltdowns." Children who do have diagnostic evaluations may be identified as having a pervasive developmental disorder not otherwise specified (PDD-NOS).

Early intervention appears to be a key to better outcomes for children on the autism spectrum, but in order to receive early intervention services, children need to be identified early. Although the average age for diagnosis of autism has moved downward, some children with autism spectrum disorders are still not identified until five or even six years of age. We now have tools such as the M-CHAT, the Modified Checklist for Autism in Toddlers (Robins et al. 2001), for screening populations of children at twenty-four months for possible autism. There are also tools for diagnosing children on the autism spectrum starting at age two or two and a half years, particularly the Autism Diagnostic Interview–Revised (Lord, Rutter, and Le Couteur 1994) and the Autism Diagnostic Observation Schedule (Lord et al. 2002). Today researchers are looking for reliable ways to identify children twelve months or younger who are likely to be diagnosed with autism by the time they are two and a half or three years old, so that services can be initiated before these children fall well behind their typically developing peers.

THE PRESCHOOL YEARS

> There is no question that the evolution of spoken language as we know it was a delivering point in human pre-history. Perhaps it was *the* defining point. Equipped with language, humans were able to create new kinds of worlds in nature: the world of introspective consciousness and the world we manufacture and share with others, which we call "culture."
>
> *(Leakey 1994, 119)*

By three years of age, most children have joined this world we share with others, and their most powerful medium for sharing is speech. Normally developing three-year-olds use speech for a variety of purposes: making their needs known, gathering information, sharing information, and directing and controlling others. The child with autism who lacks an organized system of communication has only limited entrée to this shared world.

By the time a child approaches age three and still lacks functional speech, family practitioners and pediatricians as well as parents have usually agreed on the need for a diagnostic evaluation by a specialist in childhood disorders. With federal education law mandating the provision of special education services to preschoolers with disabilities, with the availability of early intervention services to infants and toddlers with developmental delays, and with early intervention a well-advertised concept, many three-year-olds have already been diagnosed and have begun receiving special education services. The characteristic that most often drives this process is the child's lack of meaningful or functional speech. Furthermore, a critical precursor of speech, namely communicative intent, may be absent.

Communicative intent, the motivation to communicate with others, does not, in itself, ensure the development of speech or language. Some children with profound mental retardation display communicative intent but acquire only a few gestures, words, or manual signs. Communicative intent is, however, the sine qua non for functional speech. What complicates this situation is that it is difficult to differentiate a lack of communicative intent from a severe impairment in the ability to process language, to understand its function and meaning, and to organize a communicative act, whether through speech or gestures.

A lack of communicative intent is sometimes used as the central explanation for the absence of speech and gestures in preschool children with autism. The reminiscences of some adults with autism—Donna Williams and Sean Barron, for example, who recall that as children they much preferred their own worlds to the outside world—seem to support this idea. However, other adults cited in chapter 2 report very different experiences. Bill Donovan and Steffie DePaolo vividly remember their inability to produce speech in early childhood in spite of intense efforts to do so. Some young children with autism do speak, but only on rare occasions. This too is often attributed to weak motivation to communicate to others, but Temple Grandin and other adults with autism recall that their intervals without speech resulted largely from continuing, sporadic difficulty in producing speech, a problem that can be thought of as difficulty with motor planning or the organization of motor responses. In most typically developing children this is not an issue; but for some children with autism it appears to be a major hurdle, one that may be based on differences in brain structure and functioning.

The production of speech is a motor as well as a cognitive act. Even the use of gestures or signs requires the child to organize what he or she wants to communicate and to coordinate the appropriate motor actions. Difficulties can arise at any stage of this process, and children with disabilities other than autism also sometimes display motor-planning problems. A situation I observed almost thirty years ago illustrates this point. A boy of six or seven was being evaluated at a pediatric language disorder clinic. One part of this examination was a diagnostic teaching task in which the child was taught to recognize three written words and was then asked to pick them out from a small pack of word cards presented one by one. The specific directions given by the examiner were, "Stop me when you see one of these words." Twice the examiner went slowly through the pack of word cards without being stopped. Her conclusion was that the child had not learned the three words well enough to remember them and distinguish them from the other words. He had failed the task.

At that point the director of the clinic, who had been observing the evaluation, asked to take over. She gave the boy a wooden mallet from a toy workbench and instructed him, "Bang on this table hard when you see one of the words." This time the boy banged his mallet three times, once in response to each of the words he had been taught. What the first examiner had interpreted as a learning problem now appeared to be a problem in coordinating and implementing a response.

To varying degrees, motivation, cognition, and motor-planning abilities may all affect the delayed or deviant speech of individual children with autism. Slowness in organizing a response appears to be an issue that goes beyond the establishment of speech. This difficulty has been noted in verbal children and some adults with autism. Over fifty years ago, Leo Kanner, who introduced the concept of autism, told of a bright six-year-old boy with autism whose characteristic response to being asked to describe his experiences was, "Wait, I have to get it in my mind first" (1973, 91).

Language has many functions. A young child can use language to ask for attention, help, or affection; to request food or toys; to share interesting events; to protest. Both the very young child and the child who has not yet acquired a language system such as speech, sign language, or a picture communication system use prelanguage means to achieve these goals. The autistic preschooler without language may vocalize, grab, or manipulate another person's hand as if it were a tool to get food or toys. Tantrums, physical attacks, or self-injury may take the place of speech in protesting movement from favored to disliked activities or in responding to any kind of change in routines. Such prelanguage means of communication not only are often inefficient in achieving the child's objective but also create negative emotional associations between child and caregiver. They sometimes work all too well, establishing maladaptive behavior patterns such as head banging that further damage the child and limit his or her potential independence in home, school, and the larger community. For these reasons, parents and professionals should make an intensive effort to facilitate the preschool child's language development, both for understanding the communications of others and for expressing himself or herself to others. When verbal language has not become functional by the preschool years, alternative modes of communication through picture or sign language systems should be pursued along with continued efforts at developing speech.

Echolalia, or the echoing of speech, is common in autistic children who have no significant problems with the motor aspects of speech production but have difficulty understanding and using the units of speech in a meaningful way. Richard was a six-year-old with autism at a residential school who loved his psychiatrist. On Monday mornings Dr. S. came to the classroom where I taught to take Richard for his weekly "therapy" session. Referring to the boy's weekend at his family home, Dr. S. frequently asked, "Where have you been, Richard?" After a while, when Dr. S. appeared at my classroom door, Richard would say, "Where you da been Richard?" This was his reproduction of Dr. S.'s way of greeting him, and it appeared to serve both affective and communicative functions, something like "Hi, Dr. S. I'm so glad to see you again. Now let's go for our session together." Then Richard would take Dr. S.'s hand and lead him out of the classroom. Echolalia served a useful function for Richard, who could not at that time produce a spontaneous verbal expression of his happiness at seeing his psychiatrist.

Kevin, who was Richard's classmate, did have some functional speech. He made requests, was beginning to attempt simple questions, and used an emphatic "no" to decline some requests from others. Kevin also loved watching television and would periodically repeat jingles, program introductions, and closing remarks from television commercials and shows. These echolalic episodes seemed to give him pleasure while his functional speech continued to emerge and expand.

Echolalia may serve a variety of purposes for young children. It may represent a primitive attempt to communicate for children who have not been able to grasp how meaning is conveyed through language. Echolalic children may be learning language by memorizing and repeating multi-word chunks, initially with only general associations to situations or actions. Many of these children will eventually break down the chunks into smaller units and use them more appropriately. In addition, there is evidence that echolalia is more likely to occur at certain times, for example, when the child is in an unfamiliar situation. Thus, echolalia in a young child with little or no functional speech should not be viewed as pathological behavior that needs to be stamped out. Instead, we should view it as a reflection of a point in language development, recognizing the functions it may serve and offering assistance to the child in developing more appropriate expressive language. Sometimes this developmental path is clearly visible, as it was with Kenneth, the echolalic five-year-old referred to at the beginning of chapter 1. When Kenneth began to develop functional speech, his interactions often went like this:

MOTHER: "Do you want milk?"
KENNETH: "Do you want milk? Yes."

After a while, Kenneth was able to answer "yes" without first echoing his mother's question.

Even preschool children who have acquired some functional verbal language may use echolalic speech to express themselves at times, particularly when they are experiencing strong emotions. Jimmy was annoyed with his younger sister one day. He announced to his mother that "this lit-tle fart of a robot is giving me the red-ass" (Fling 2000, 36). That statement was taken verbatim from Jimmy's favorite movie, in which a character used those words to express anger at a robot. Echo Fling, Jimmy's mother, explained to a psychologist who was going to test Jimmy:

> "Jimmy has a very hard time communicating his thoughts," I said. "Unless you have the benefit of seeing his favorite video, you rarely have any idea of what he is trying to say. . . . By the time he gets it clear in his mind what he wants to say, the rest of the world is two conversa-tion topics ahead," I said. "Or worse, he takes too long and totally breaks down altogether and forgets what it was he was thinking about in the first place. . . ." This makes it very hard for him to carry on a normal con-versation with other children, who are much, much quicker with things like this. (Fling 2000, 63)

Not all children with autism develop echolalia. Some acquire only a handful of word approximations. In the past, about 50 percent of indi-viduals with autism failed to develop functional speech. With the em-phasis on early identification and intervention since the late 1980s, and the intensification of educational services to infants, toddlers, and preschoolers with autism or other pervasive developmental disorders beginning in the 1990s, this percentage has declined significantly. A recent book by the director of the autism center clinic at the University of California, Santa Barbara, states that "today about 90% of children with autism are able to learn to use words and language to communicate, if intervention starts before age five" (Koegel and LaZebnik 2004, 40).

When a young child with autism responds appropriately to a spoken request, the child may be using cues other than words to guide his or her responses. This occurs most often in the context of common routines, where speech may serve primarily as an alerting signal. Thus, a young boy may respond appropriately to his mother's request to "Come here now; it's time to work," even though he doesn't understand her words. What may be guiding his response is the routine of his mother being seated at a particular table with his chair facing hers, a situation that occurs several times each afternoon. Understanding speech involves breaking the stream of speech sounds into discrete units in accordance with the rules of a particular language. To autistic children who haven't cracked the language code, speech may be a continuous flow of sounds, an undifferentiated chunk of stimuli punctuated by periods of silence.

When communications are too complex for the young autistic child to understand, even with the assistance of situational cues, the child may well tune out the speech addressed to him or her. Sometimes adults interpret this tuning out as the child's refusal to follow directions. This situation can escalate into a destructive interaction between the child and the caregiver, with the adult becoming insistent and angry and the child becoming anxious and perhaps engaging in aggressive or self-injurious behavior. To minimize such interactions, parents, teachers, and others must understand the child's level of language comprehension and use language well within that range. The exception to this general rule is carefully planned instruction targeted at expanding language skills, which pushes at the boundaries of the child's current level of language comprehension.

While young children with autism have severe difficulty with most aspects of language, a small number of preschoolers with autism learn to read or at least to recite words correctly from the written page, often with little or no formal instruction, to the amazement of their parents and teachers. A three-year-old with no speech, who made few attempts at communicating with others, was observed using plastic letters to form words that he had previously seen on the television screen. At age four, after he had learned to name some objects, this boy would identify the words he had constructed with his letters. Visual-spatial skills and visual memory are areas of strength for many children with autism. Hyperlexia, or early reading not expected on the basis of IQ or language development, reflects these strengths.

The term "hyperlexia" once carried some negative connotations. In the past some professionals denigrated this ability in various ways, perceiving it as a rote skill that had no functional value. That view has changed as professionals recognized that such early, unexpected reading was often more than just word naming and that even when the child's comprehension of the words being read was poor, this skill might be beneficial. Freed from the need to teach word recognition, teachers can concentrate on developing better comprehension in these children. In fact, hyperlexia appears to be associated with better developmental outcomes. Moreover, early reading provides the young child who has autism with a skill easily recognized by typical peers, a situation that can work to the child's advantage when he or she is included in such mainstream settings as preschool, kindergarten, or first grade.

While some infants and toddlers with autism appear to look through people, treat them as tools, and fail to recognize their parents, by age three or four most children with autism have begun to relate to selected others—one or both parents, a sibling, and perhaps a grandparent. Clara Park describes this change in her daughter Jessy. At age two Jessy appeared for the most part to look at her parents and siblings "as through a pane of glass." By the time she was three her "flashes of response" had become more frequent, and her indifference to her mother had turned into "a kind of attachment," with Jessy following her mother from room to room (1986, 83–84). What remains distinctive about the behavior of preschool children with autism, even when compared to mentally retarded children, is their lack of interest in other children and their odd, impoverished play.

Normally developing toddlers who are brought together are likely to make social overtures to one another. They may smile, offer a toy, or take a toy. While playing separately, they may have occasional brief interactions. By age four play changes markedly, with cooperative play common and make-believe play dominating children's joint endeavors. Preschoolers engage in pretend play themes of cooking and eating, doing housework and shopping, being firefighters or bus drivers or doctors, and being sick. At the same age children with autism are likely to ignore peers, and their version of play is likely to be repetitive, inflexible manipulation of objects and object parts—lining them up, spinning them, or diddling with them.

A variety of explanations have been suggested to account for the distinctive play pattern of children with autism. Given the fact that many young autistic children have little or no language and develop slowly in other areas as well, we might attribute play differences to these developmental delays. But these distinctions in play patterns have been found even in studies that have compared children with autism to other children with similar mental ages and language abilities. Several researchers offer another explanation, namely that children with autism have difficulty overriding the reality-based features of their environment and shifting to internal representations not closely tied to these features, a process basic to make-believe play. In pretend play a doll is a baby, and that baby is fed with a bottle that contains no milk; a child has a conversation with someone on a toy telephone when no one is on the other end; the child goes to "sleep" while actually awake and not in bed. Pretend play has an "as if" quality. It veers from the here-and-now reality of the child's situation. Most preschool children can make this shift easily and enjoy doing so. Young autistic children appear to have difficulty with this process of engaging in play schemes not tied to their immediate situations.

Another factor may also be relevant here. The play of young children is based to a large extent on imitation of actions performed by others, either in past situations or in the present. Imitation, which is a fundamental mode of learning, appears to be an ability that some children with autism don't develop naturally. They have to be taught this skill, which normally developing infants exhibit.

Preschool children who have developed verbal language and who are later labeled as having Asperger syndrome also have unusual play patterns. They appear to lack interest in interactive play with their peers and in the typical subjects of preschoolers' dramatic play. Instead, they pursue interests in specific, narrow subjects in a solitary fashion, occasionally responding to an adult's attempt to make their play more interactive by citing facts that they have accumulated. And these interests may be quite unusual, for example, vacuum cleaners, drains, fans, traffic lights, locks. At age five, in his third year of preschool, Jimmy still had difficulty socializing at school, Echo Fling tells us. Her son still hadn't made any friends and couldn't tell his mother the name of a single child in his class. Nor did this seem to bother him.

During the preschool years stereotyped movements may become more frequent. During the toddler period spinning, rocking, and walking in circles might have been noted. By age three hand flapping, finger flicking, and pacing back and forth may become prominent. These odd movements, which do not serve any clearly apparent function, may make other children and their parents uncomfortable, thus contributing to the isolation of many children with autism. However, adults with autism spectrum disorders tell us that these stereotyped movements often serve an important function: they release tension arising from the stress of dealing with an overwhelming and confusing environment.

Problems with hypersensitivity to sensory stimulation do not disappear by the preschool years, and sometimes they have an unrecognized connection to negative relationships within the family. Jimmy's father was upset. He felt that Jimmy didn't like him and was pushing him out of his life. Jimmy virtually ignored his father but was responsive to his mother. A closer look at this situation revealed that the problem was the bombardment of stimulation presented by Jimmy's father, who would grab his son, give him a big hug, ruffle his hair, and talk to him loudly. In contrast, Jimmy's mother would invite him to give her a hug and sit quietly with her hands at her side while Jimmy leaned on her and gave her a sort of snuggle. Within three weeks of the time that Jimmy's father started imitating his wife's behavior, Jimmy became more responsive to him (Fling 2000, 149).

The mother of a preschool girl who would later be diagnosed as having Asperger syndrome described her puzzlement about her daughter's behavior:

> "I can't put my finger on it, but Mere seems lost. She is doing well in school. She has a friend or two. She has toys she enjoys. She follows the rules and seems very capable of organizing her things and tending to business. In fact, she is the most tenacious kid I know. Once she sets her mind to something, look out! In fact, Lord help those of us who do not follow the rules or do not appreciate the thing she is interested in. But, well . . . it just does not fit. She's just not like other kids!" I would write in my journal, "Look at her. Watch her. Don't you see? Something is different. Something's going on. What can it be? What can it be . . . ?" (Willey 2002, 14)

Until Mere was six years old, the cues for Asperger syndrome were missed or misinterpreted by everyone other than her mother, even by the family doctor, who was himself the father of a boy with autistic disorder. As a three-year-old, Mere could talk and could play with another child, so, observers asked, how could she have a pervasive developmental disorder? They were, however, overlooking the rigid routines, the aloofness from classmates most of the time, and the intensive interests that Mere expected her peers to share. Asperger syndrome is often not diagnosed until after age five.

Before turning to the middle years of childhood let's meet a young boy, Ned Christopher, whose early years seemed very promising, and then check back on Tony Callahan, whose early years, described at the beginning of this chapter, had seemed less so. Many TV viewers knew Ned's father, William Christopher, as Father Mulcahy of *M*A*S*H*. What these viewers did not know was that his (adopted) son Ned was diagnosed at age three as having atypical development with autistic features. Yet to his parents and some professionals, Ned's disability seemed very mild, in spite of some unusual behavior.

> "Did you ever hear of a kid who didn't like piggyback?" said his frustrated father. No, he didn't like piggyback, just as he hadn't liked being cuddled when he was a tiny infant. He hadn't liked it, and he had stiffened his little body into a board, making it impossible to cuddle him. (Christopher and Christopher 1989, 12)

But before age three Ned could write the letters of the alphabet, was trying to dress himself independently, and demanded to be told the name of every flag he saw by shouting "flag." He rocked in bed as he slept, but he could recognize and name vegetables and plants in the yard and neighborhood. He didn't respond to strangers who said "Hi" or asked what his name was, but he could count to forty. By age three he could spell and read about fifty words, but he had begun to pull the hair of the little girls in his nursery school class, which was the only time he interacted with any of his classmates. A regular kindergarten class was the goal at that point. In the meantime Ned spent mornings in a special education program with a behavioral approach and continued afternoons in a nursery school. By the end of that year a regular kindergarten program no longer appeared to be a possibility. Shortly before Ned turned six his mother wrote: "Even though his language, behavior, abilities all move forward, it just isn't coming together. . . . Perhaps it is that as he grows older, the gap between Ned and a normal child becomes more obvious" (Christopher and Christopher 1989, 69).

Tony's progress through the preschool years was quite different. By age four, prodded and instructed by his younger sister, Renee, Tony had begun to engage in dramatic play and conversation. Renee and Tony were playing at giving "juice" to a doll when the following conversation occurred:

RENEE: I spill it.
TONY: No spilling it.
RENEE: I have to.
TONY: You don't have to.
RENEE: Yea, I have to.
TONY: No, you don't have to.
RENEE: Yea.
TONY: No, you don't have to.
RENEE: I have to (screaming).
TONY: I be mad at you. (Callahan 1987, 118)

At age five, with more than a year in a special preschool program, Tony was still not talking to his classmates; he didn't understand them, he told his mother. After months of work on auditory processing with his mother, Tony entered a regular kindergarten class; the school staff knew nothing about his earlier diagnosis of autism. Six weeks later his anxious mother, afraid of what she would learn the following day at a parent-teacher conference, asked the teacher aide how Tony was doing. "'Tony?' she responded with a puzzled look. 'He's doing great. I wish we had a classroom full of kids like Tony. Why?'" (Callahan 1987, 164).

These two children illustrate the different developmental pathways or trajectories that autism may follow. They represent hope and fear for the future. More and more children today follow the upward path of Tony, but for reasons still not completely clear, some do not.

MIDDLE CHILDHOOD

Nellie was again biting her already callused hand. She made noises that sounded like anger. I was new to working with children like Nellie, having previously taught kindergarten and first grade in a public school. I tried to protect Nellie from herself, to take her hand from her mouth. When I finally succeeded, her jaws closed forcefully on my thumb. I struggled to extract it. Her resistance and power astonished me. Nellie was a small girl of six and a half, but I feared that I would not see that thumb in one piece again. After a couple of minutes Nellie relaxed her jaw slightly, and I managed to extract my thumb, damaged but still whole.

For most children the middle childhood years are a time of expansion, of moving into the world of formal education and the world of peers; a time for hard work and close friendships. For some children with autism the years from five or six to about twelve are a period of learning and expansion as well, but during the early part of this time span diverging paths become apparent, one pointing toward the possibility of higher, near-normal functioning, the other with an unclear end point but with a much greater likelihood of continued significant disability.

Nellie seemed to be on this second path. She rarely spoke and then only in single words or short phrases that voiced demands, usually for food. During Nellie's preschool years her limited and infrequent communication had not seemed to be as serious a problem as it did now, and her hands had not yet become callused from being bitten. At age six these behaviors began to seem much more deviant. Together with the limited progress she had made during the previous year, they damaged her family's hopes for her future as well as the optimism of the professional team responsible for her treatment.

Self-abusive behavior is not uncommon in individuals with autism, although it is not characteristic of most autistic children or adults. During the middle childhood years both self-injurious behavior and aggression toward others may become more apparent and more difficult to cope with or control. Head banging has been noted in normally developing infants and toddlers, as well as in babies who are later diagnosed as autistic. In normally developing young children, this behavior occurs mostly at bedtime and disappears altogether before age three; whereas in some autistic children, head banging may occur at various times of the day during varied activities and may increase as the child gets older.

A variety of reasons have been proposed to explain this behavior, including the attention and concern it gains the child, the escape from disliked activities it achieves, and the sensory stimulation it provides. Head banging or other types of self-injury sometimes accompany painful medical problems such as severe earaches, which the autistic child with little functional language has no way of reporting. Neurochemical disturbances, particularly dysfunctions in neurotransmitter systems, have also been proposed as causing or contributing to self-injurious behavior. Frontal lobe seizures are another hypothesized cause of self-injury in some individuals with autism, although there is no hard evidence to back up this theory.

When six-year-old Sean was placed in my class, his forehead was bumpy and bruised. During the first few weeks, I feared for his vision because he banged his head against the glass windows many times, and I anticipated that one day the glass would break from the force of those blows. I don't know what motivated this self-abuse: perhaps fear, perhaps his inability to communicate his needs, perhaps in part the concern his behavior generated. Whatever the cause, his head banging declined dramatically after a while as other behaviors emerged. Sean and I played interactive infant games like variants of peek-a-boo, and he giggled when my face reappeared. He imitated my block stacking, and we both laughed when the stacks fell down. Sean began calling me something that resembled "ma ma" when he wanted my attention. Still, one day when he entered the classroom and tripped on his untied shoelace, Sean began to bang his head against the floor. Was this anthropomorphic thinking? Did Sean think the floor had tripped him, or was he flailing out against the pain of a world he did not understand?

Self-injurious behavior can become entrenched and difficult to eliminate. Yet with skilled intervention, self-injury can be significantly reduced in almost all children with autism. In the last fifteen years or so, a whole system of functional behavioral analysis has evolved for identifying the factors that may precipitate or maintain self-injurious behavior and for designing treatment strategies to eliminate it. Medication may need to be part of the treatment package in selected cases, although it should be noted that medication may sometimes trigger or increase self-injury.

To parents and teachers tantrums or meltdowns are one of the most troubling behaviors exhibited by children with autism spectrum disorders. They limit activities outside the home, increase family tensions, and interfere with inclusion of the child in the mainstream of school. Temper tantrums are common in typically developing two-year-olds, but by the preschool years they become less frequent and less ominous in most children. This is often not the case in regard to children with autism.

> I tell him about the temper tantrum Jonah had today. He tried to bite me in the parking lot, then threw a crying fit when I refused to play his Barney music as punishment. . . . "I didn't tell you about the second tantrum he had in the bathroom when we came home. I took his hat and water gun away so he would pee, and he pitched a fit. He threw himself down and tried to throw things. It scared me." (Adams 2005, 244)

Meltdowns may continue in the middle years, when the aggression that is sometimes part of them may be viewed as quite serious. The trigger for these meltdowns is often a change in environment or routine. Children with autism appear to have an overwhelming need for sameness. Echo Fling gives us an example:

> One time I changed the picture arrangement in our living room and he got violent. It was the first (and only time) he had ever hit me. Although he was a seven-year-old, Jimmy's whack across my back really hurt me. I had no clue why he had such a strong reaction to the new pictures. . . . I began to cry in front of my son. He was astonished. . . . I was simply sobbing my eyes out. In part because my back smarted, on the other part, my heart was broken. To think that my own son could do this to me. Immediate thoughts of his future flooded my eyes through the tears. Children who grow up hitting their mothers are residents of our local jails. (Fling 2000, 136)

A major shift in mental functioning occurs between ages five and seven or eight in most children. By the end of this period language has become their vehicle of thought, and their thinking has become more logical. At this time, too, children become much more skilled at recognizing the codes of social behavior and acting in accordance with them. Children with autism spectrum disorders who have acquired functional language by the early part of this period can apply their energies to academic achievement and to learning the rules of social behavior. Autistic children who have not learned to understand speech and to express themselves through speech or another language system are likely to make slow progress in most areas of development during this same time period.

> The autistic child presents a singular puzzle: a human being whose conversational language and social skills generally lag way behind apparent intellectual ability. Everywhere else one looks in the human domain, even among those with low IQ, social contact and conversational fluency seem to develop so effortlessly that it looks as if they required no particular skill at all. (Bruner and Feldman 1993, 273)

In the middle childhood years the wide diversity within the autism population becomes strikingly apparent. While some children are still nonverbal, others have acquired large vocabularies; while some still appear unable to understand speech that would make sense to most toddlers, others seem to have nearly age-appropriate language comprehension. Some children with autism learn to read as preschoolers, perhaps with only limited comprehension of what they are reading; others may understand written language, as shown by their ability to answer questions based on the written text, even though they do not speak. Whatever their differences in acquiring language, one area of communication in which most children with autism spectrum disorders show poor skills is conversation. They may be able to talk, but they can't converse.

Conducting a conversation is something most children learn to do with little formal instruction. Parents and teachers of preschoolers may have to say, "Wait your turn" or "Give someone else a turn," from time to time, and occasionally an adult may be heard coaching a child with a phrase such as "Why don't you ask him about what he watched on television yesterday?" But these kinds of casual reminders in natural situations are all the instruction most young children need. Yet children with autism may need instruction in a range of skills involved in conducting conversations, including how to identify a suitable topic; start a conversation; attend to what the other person is saying; respond to what the other person is saying; take turns; use appropriate gestures, facial expressions, and proximity; and end a conversation.

Although children with Asperger syndrome might be verbally fluent, they often lack skills at a more subtle level. They may use signals inappropriately to indicate the intended recipient of their communication. Some begin a conversation without adequately introducing their topic or by making incorrect assumptions about what the partner in the conversation knows or is interested in. They may fail to recognize when it is time to relinquish their turn because they cannot "read" the nonverbal signals from their partner. Their tendency to talk incessantly about one particular topic of interest to them can drive away possible friends. Repetition is attractive to many individuals with autism spectrum disorders, who repeat the same questions over and over again both at school and at home.

Pragmatics—the use of language appropriate to the social context and the goal of the communicative exchange—has been identified as problematic for children with Asperger syndrome. Pragmatics involves principles of communication that are widely understood, some of them even by typical preschoolers. Preschoolers tailor their speech to the ages of their listeners: when addressing younger children, they speak in shorter, simpler sentences than they use when they talk to older children or adults. Preschoolers also modify the information they communicate depending on how well they know the listener and whether the listener has had direct contact with the subject of the conversation. School-age children with Asperger syndrome and other autism spectrum disorders, however, often do not modify their communications according to the context and identity of the listener. Obviously, problems can arise when a child in an elementary school talks to the school principal and to classmates in the same way.

Friendships become very important in the middle childhood years, but most children with autism don't form close relationships with peers during this period. One of the reasons why this may be so is that most children with autism spectrum disorders appear to lack or be slow in developing a faculty referred to as *theory of mind*, that is, the capacity to understand mental states—for example, beliefs, intentions, feelings, hopes, pretense—and to interpret behavior in terms of such mental states. Since this ability appears in all typically developing children without explicit teaching, it is considered an innate capacity or mechanism governed by a particular part of the brain. The absence of this ability to understand what people know, think, and feel may be at the root of some of the difficulties that individuals with autism spectrum disorders have in communication and relationships. We can make sense of the behavior of others because we can think about their thinking and therefore anticipate their responses to various situations and interactions. Richard Leakey (1994) identifies this ability to predict the behavior of others as the central challenge for individuals in primate society. To a child with autism who cannot take into consideration how others are likely to feel, think, or react, the social world must be a perplexing and terrifying place in which to exist—a message that several adults with autism communicated to us in chapter 2.

During middle childhood, many children with autism start seeking out other children. One mother reported the following episode after her son had invited another boy to his home to play:

> There they were outside on the swing set and the next time I looked up, he was in his room lining up figures, and the friend was just left sitting on the swing set. He had no idea that it wasn't cool to do that, even though we talked about it 100 times. (Church and Coplan 1995, 27)

This behavior reflects the tenuous connection of many children with autism to their peers and illustrates the theory of mind deficit that may, at least to some degree, underlie it. A theory of mind deficit may also be responsible for the naïveté observed in many children with autism, reflecting an inability to read intentions, as illustrated by this example:

> Samantha, a ten-year-old girl with autism attending a mainstream school, was deliberately teased by the children there, and frequently they would tell her to perform some unacceptable act, such as taking her clothes off in the playground. She was quite bewildered by the laughter that ensued . . . believing that her compliance would result in them becoming "her friend." (Baron-Cohen and Howlin 1993, 467)

Similarly, the long monologues of some children, adolescents, and adults with autism that cause the persons they are addressing to seek escape may result from an inability to sense their listeners' level of interest; and the embarrassment or hurt that individuals with autism sometimes inflict on others may stem from an inability to anticipate how their comments will affect other people.

> One young man . . . complained that he couldn't "mind-read." He went on to explain that other people seemed to have a special sense by which they could read other people's thoughts and could anticipate their responses and feelings; he knew this because they managed to avoid upsetting people whereas he was always putting his foot in it, not realizing that he was doing or saying the wrong thing until after the other person became angry or upset. (Rutter 1983, 526)

What is accomplished by giving a name—theory of mind—to a capacity that appears to be underdeveloped in many individuals with autism? The processes of prevention and treatment are shaped by understanding; and understanding of core or primary characteristics of autism may both lead to improved treatment and illuminate the search for the neurobiological factors underlying this condition. Is a theory of mind deficit a core characteristic of autism? For well over a decade researchers have explored this question. Somewhere between 40 and 80 percent of autistic children can't predict the beliefs of others on the same tests passed by typically developing and mentally retarded children of similar mental ages, although most children with autism spectrum disorders improve in this ability over time. Thus, at the present time the construct of a theory of mind deficit in autism appears to be a useful way of looking at and studying some of the difficulties in interactive communication and social relationships experienced by individuals with autism. A few years from now, after we learn more about autism, we may identify more productive ways of viewing these difficulties.

A theoretical construct used to explain other types of problems that many children with autism spectrum disorders exhibit in school and home is *executive function*. Executive function refers to higher-level abilities such as planning, inhibition, mental flexibility, and organization, which are important when dealing with complex situations. A child may be quite bright but also be unable to develop an appropriate plan to address a problem, to inhibit irrelevant thoughts that interfere with problem solving, or to organize the materials needed to attack the problem. Executive function problems are common in children with Asperger syndrome and children with attention-deficit/hyperactivity disorder (ADHD).

Middle childhood is also the period when the special abilities of some autistic children become very apparent. A parent described the skill her son had developed at age five in opening locks:

> When our son was about five, he had exceptional skill with locks. . . .
> One day we took him to the grocery store that happened to have a large safe. It immediately drew his attention. I told my son to get away from the lock. However, the clerk intervened to say that it was okay for him to play with it because it was an expensive burglar-proof safe that he couldn't damage. . . .
> I think I made it through the first aisle before the alarms went off as the huge safe door began to swing open. Both the clerk and the store manager stood there with their mouths open. (Gilpin 1994, 30–31)

By the age of six some children with autism know the routes to multiple distant destinations. Others display amazing "calendar skills," remembering the day and date of events that occurred months earlier, figuring out the day of the week of events that occurred before they were born or that will occur in the future, or being skilled at various other processes involving numbers. "Bobby" was one such child. His therapist writes of this five-year-old boy who had not yet begun school or had any formal instruction:

> Although his speech was still idiosyncratic and it was still common for him to run up and down, flapping his arms, he was now able to read, sounding out any words he didn't know; he could add and subtract; his memory was phenomenal; and he could remember many telephone numbers and addresses, as well as the complete New York City bus and subway systems! He could also remember the dates on which events occurred. (Pinney and Schlachter 1983, 233).

A few months later, when Bobby was six, he spent a month in London with his therapist, who had returned there. She notes: "By the time he left he knew by heart the entire London Underground and all the bus routes; sometimes sitting up until three o'clock in the morning, surrounded by pieces of paper, mapping these details and noting the connections" (238). Furthermore, Bobby could apply this information, although still in ways that may have seemed odd if not bizarre, as another adult reports:

> He would stand by the sliding doors; he would announce to the people inside the train what station we had reached and what lines intersected at that station. He would then, when the doors had opened, announce to the people standing outside where the train was going and what lines it would intersect with further along the route. (Pinney and Schlachter 1983, 240)

The developmental psychologist Howard Gardner has proposed a theory of multiple intelligences, which he has presented in publications such as the books *Frames of Mind* (1983) and *Multiple Intelligences* (1993). The functioning of people with autism was important in the formation of this theory. While children with autism generally have very poor linguistic or verbal skills, which are commonly equated with intelligence, a substantial number of autistic children undoubtedly have superior ability in the area that Gardner calls spatial intelligence. Other children with autism excel at what Gardner refers to as logical-mathematical intelligence or at what he calls musical intelligence.

During middle childhood the term "higher-functioning," as in higher-functioning autism, begins to be used frequently in regard to children with autistic disorder who acquire speech and do grade-level academic work in most areas. But the use of this term overlooks some children who have excellent cognitive abilities but have not been able to acquire speech. Several examples of such individuals come to mind, but the one I will describe is a nine-year-old boy who is in the ninth grade of a virtual high school. At a recent conference his mother, Morton Ann Gernsbacher, a psycholinguist who has devoted herself to her son's development, described some of her son's abilities. All of his communications and school work are done on a computer. He has successfully completed a curriculum through grade eight and is taking an honors course in English. He started an extracurricular book club, for which he wrote book reviews. He designed custom t-shirts with *Sesame Street* characters for John Kerry's presidential campaign. He participates fully in the discussion boards of his high school classes, and he has online conversations with a girl in his ninth grade class about various topics of interest to both of them, such as boating.

There is nothing wrong with the theory of mind skills of Morton Ann Gernsbacher's son. When she was about to tell him that he had to organize the "stuff" in his room that was spread out all over the floor, he wrote to her: "I think it's funny how you're now trying to think of ways to organize my stuff. Give it up. It's futile" (Gernsbacher 2005). A theme heard throughout this conference from both medical researchers and parents was the uniqueness of individual children with autism. It's time to start looking more closely from a research perspective at individual differences among children identified as having autism spectrum disorders; and it's time to stop rejecting ideas because they don't apply to most children with what may turn out to be the multiple conditions we now refer to as autism.

"How is my son doing?" a father asks rhetorically in the introduction to his second book about his then eleven-year-old autistic child. "He is doing better than he has done, but not as well as I would have hoped. If I had once seen his malady as transient, I now know it to be permanent. . . . And as for Noah's future—I prefer not to think about it" (Greenfeld 1978, 3).

That was the future for one father. Other fathers have brighter prospects.

ADOLESCENCE AND YOUNG ADULTHOOD

In a 1995 letter appealing for contributions, the Autism Society of America reported the following story from a parent of a young adult with autism:

Last week, I was shopping for a winter coat for my daughter, Stephanie. While we were trying on coats something upset her terribly. Stephanie, who is eighteen and has autism, threw herself on the floor and started kicking, crying, and screaming at the top of her lungs. I pleaded with her to tell me why she was so upset, but nothing I could do would calm her down. Stephanie's tantrum was wreaking havoc. The sales clerks and customers were staring and whispering and I even heard one woman criticizing my parenting skills.

I wanted to yell to that woman, "Put yourself in my shoes! I'm doing my best here. . . . "

Adolescence can bring an exacerbation of continuing problems and the appearance of new ones. Aggressive behavior that continues from childhood may become more disruptive and dangerous. A small proportion of autistic adolescents have seizures for the first time, and the seizures may be associated with behavioral deterioration—more rituals, compulsions, and acting out. Some adolescents with milder forms of autism become aware of their social limitations and are greatly distressed by them. Depression may ensue.

New problems accompanied Ned Christopher's approaching adolescence. Ned began having outbursts of aggressive behavior in which he attacked his mother, pulling at her and pinching her until she was covered with bruises. More and more he appeared to be in an agitated state, and soon he began lashing out at others. After almost a year of professional help of various kinds that accomplished little, Ned was moved out of his family home. It took six more years of consultation with some of the best professionals in California before Ned's aggressive behavior seemed to fade, but the promise of his early years did not return.

In contrast, the screeching, hitting, biting, and tantrums of many children with autism stop or decrease significantly by adolescence, and their rigidity loosens up enough to make everyday living less stressful for them and more tolerable for the family. Some youngsters with autism have achieved near-normal functioning by adolescence and are doing well in school. They may no longer meet criteria for autism, although they might still need some special supports at school and more supportive guidance at home. Others, while still recognized as having autism, may become more socially oriented and make progress in academic work while developing greater independence in everyday functioning. The special abilities of some adolescents with autism in such areas as art, music, mathematics, science, or computer science may receive wider recognition and continue to develop during these years.

Special abilities, however, do not necessarily go hand in hand with higher functioning in other areas. Clara Park's daughter Jessy, described in chapter 1, showed giftedness in mathematics as well as great skill in art. But in adolescence and young adulthood, some of her thinking was like that of a child, in spite of an IQ in the average range. She had great difficulty, for example, in dealing with language on anything but a literal level. In her early twenties, Jessy was working at understanding proverbs, a major project for her. In trying to master the proverb "Don't cross that bridge until you come to it," she asked: "Does it mean go over the bridge or go under?" And in applying this proverb to a real situation, when she thought the family cat was lost but it later showed up, she said: "And there wasn't any bridge!" Some months later when Jessy caught herself obsessing about threatening clouds, she said: "It would be crossing the bridge too early—I would fall into the water" (Park 1986, 95).

Literalness in language is a characteristic commonly found in children and adolescents with autism. It is also a characteristic common in typical children below age five or six, but by age seven most children understand that words may be used in different ways to express different meanings, and they absorb those meanings without specific instruction. Not so in the case of many children and adolescents with autism spectrum disorders.

> After several years of hard work with my son Michael, he was finally doing fairly well fitting into the community.
>
> For his eleventh birthday I took him with me to the bakery to let him order his cake himself, with the cartoon characters he preferred. He did real well answering questions like what flavor, color frosting, filling. . . . You could tell he was losing patience, though, when the lady asked him what he wanted the cake to say.
>
> He glanced up at her and said, "Are you crazy! Cakes can't talk!"
> (Gilpin 1993, 4–5)

Another parent's tale of literal language is as follows:

> Our family Saturday project was to scrub oil spills off the driveway. I'd just gotten started when I had to go back inside for another bucket of water. When I returned, I found my son, who has autism, scrubbing merrily away while he was holding his face close to the stain and yelling at the top of his lungs. At first I was totally confused, until I noticed the detergent we were using, Shout. You've guessed it, he was following their slogan and was trying to "Shout it out!" (Gilpin 1994, 62)

Ted, a young adult with autism who had overcome most of his communication problems, also treated words literally. When his mother asked him the meaning of "a bum steer," a phrase he had read aloud from a billboard, Ted replied: "That's a cow without a job." He became quite upset at the ensuing laughter. It turned out that on an earlier occasion Ted had asked someone about this billboard and had been answered with the pun he had just repeated. He had not recognized that the response he had received was meant as humor (Hart 1989, 278). Ted, in fact, wanted very much to have a sense of humor but couldn't grasp the basic characteristics of humor, the qualities of jokes that make them funny. He worked at it, creating "knock, knock" jokes like the following: "Knock, knock." "Who's there?" "Ms." "Ms. who?" "Ms. Brutal Gorilla!" He would follow his joke with the question, "Funny?" (288). Ted couldn't tell what others would find humorous.

For many individuals with autistic disorder, adolescents and adults as well as children, nothing about language comes easily. It's almost as if an innate capacity of humans to acquire language naturally is damaged or missing, and every aspect of language has to be learned separately through deliberate study. Even when people with autistic disorder are strongly motivated and work hard, as Jessy Park and Ted Hart did, the process of developing language skills can be painstakingly slow.

I met Melvin P. at a conference of a state association on autism. He had been singled out to receive an award for his accomplishments. He was a student at a junior college who had good course grades that he achieved by dint of very hard work. He read a brief speech of thanks for the award and returned to his seat, searching his mother's face for feedback on how he had done. When the session ended people were standing around talking, and I noticed that Melvin P. was standing alone. I introduced myself to him and began a conversation.

"Mr. P., I was happy to hear that you're doing so well at college." *[A long time passes with no response even though Mr. P. is looking at me. I again attempt to initiate a conversation, this time providing a question that should be easy for him to answer.]*

"What courses are you taking at college?"

"Computers. I'm a computer major." *[Long pause]*

"How many credits are there in that program?"

"I don't know." *[Long pause]*

"What other kinds of courses do you take?"

"Math. Communications." *[Long pause]*

"Is the semester over?"

"It ended on May 18." *[Long pause]*

"Are you going to summer school?"

"I'm going again in September. I have to ask my counselor how many credits the program has." *[Long pause]*

"How many credits did you take this semester?"

"Twelve. Thank you for talking to me."

At that point Melvin P. seemed to need a break from the effort involved in his role in the conversation. It was none too soon; I too needed a break from the effort my role had involved. The long pauses in the conversation occurred because I was waiting for Mr. P. to elaborate on his short factual responses, or ask me a question, or introduce a new idea, all strategies for maintaining a conversation. Engaging in small talk is something individuals with autism find very challenging. I wondered about his conversations with peers, who were very likely of greater interest to him but who could not be counted on to keep supplying him with questions. Could Mr. P. maintain a conversation without being cued by questions? Could he contribute enough to a conversation to engage the interest of other young adults who were not autistic? Could he "mind-read" them well enough to tell when someone was interested?

Thomas was a thirteen-year-old with Asperger syndrome. His greatest difficulty was dealing with peers at junior high school. This was a new problem. In the sixth grade, he had been accepted and popular with his classmates, who enjoyed his special type of humor. Now he was socially isolated although he wanted to have friends. His mother reported that when he started noticing girls he realized that he had a hard time socializing; and he felt bad about not knowing how to talk to other boys or girls when everyone else seemed to know how to do that.

Jay was a fifteen-year-old with Asperger syndrome. He too had a strong wish for friends but did not have any, despite his attempts: "He kind of goes through this obsession thing, where he picks one person and he decides that he wants that person as a friend, and he kind of smothers that person. . . . But he doesn't understand how to small talk, so it's hard for him to make friends" (Marks et al. 2000, 10).

The end of schooling, which comes at age twenty-one for most individuals with autism, often marks the beginning of a difficult transition period. Everyday routines are disrupted, and any major change is stressful to people with autism. There is also the question of what is to take the place of school. Although many individuals with Asperger syndrome go on to college, that is not the case for most individuals with autistic disorder, and few can move into jobs independently. Since 1991 transition planning has been a required component of educational programs for older adolescents with significant disabilities. When school programs and state-supported programs for adults with developmental disabilities are well coordinated, a twenty-one-year-old with autistic disorder will move into a work-oriented training program followed by a supported work program in the community. Unfortunately, significant problems frequently occur in this process, and the movement to work is rarely smooth.

The other issue that often arises at about this point in the lives of individuals with autism is where they will live. By the time the person with autism reaches young adulthood, most parents and other family caregivers are totally exhausted. Some parents may be approaching their late years, with their energies and health deteriorating. Others may feel that after twenty-one years, they need a chance to experience the freedom common to other parents whose children have grown up. Thus, many families begin to look for another place or another way of living for their son or daughter. While many supervised and supported living alternatives have become available since the 1980s, making a good match between the needs or desires of the individual with autism and the family on the one hand and the available residential arrangements on the other frequently proves to be a time-consuming and stressful process.

I visited a group home and work program for adults with autism. The agency providing these services was operated by two members of the family of an autistic man. I had first met one member of this team many years earlier, when we were both on an advisory panel on services for siblings of individuals with developmental disabilities. This sibling served as my guide.

Our starting point was a retail shop that featured handicrafts by autistic adults, in addition to other items. The adults producing these items were at work in one section of the shop. Scattered about the store were tiny signs reading, YOUR PURCHASE HELPS OUR AUTISTIC YOUNG ADULTS TO BE PRODUCTIVE . . . AND EMPLOYED. *It was close to Christmas, so many of the products featured reflected that seasonal theme — decorated wreaths and linens embroidered with Christmas motifs. Also displayed were items not tied to the seasons, like note cards. I bought a box of these cards, drawn by their charming young look and humor. Marshall, the brother of my guide, was the artist on several of them. He is a productive person; for five hours each day he works at tasks involved in creating various items for sale. Marshall still sometimes exhibits behavior that causes stress to people who love him and may frighten some people who don't. Although he usually communicates through speech, at times when he's very upset he might make sounds like loud barking and hit his thigh with his clenched hands. During my visit I happened to witness one such episode. Afterward Marshall took my hand and stroked it while telling me about computer games he liked — almost as if he wanted to make sure I experienced the gentle, loving side that's very much a part of him. I wondered if Marshall had Tourette syndrome as well as autism.*

It's easy, when you focus on young children as I had been doing, to fall into the trap of thinking that if only autistic children could achieve language and communication, they would be on their way to near-normal functioning. Not so, the adults I saw in the shop reminded me. Language is a critical achievement, but language alone doesn't turn autistic children into nonautistic adults. There are other fundamental differences in functioning, and significant problems continue to distinguish most adults with autism from "typicals." The nine adults in the shop all spoke; however, how they spoke and what they said were still quite unusual.

Daniel, a man I met there, was in his forties and lived in an apartment with another autistic man as his roommate, under the supervision of the agency providing the services and programs I observed. Daniel's need for control over his environment had taken on an obsessive-compulsive quality. Not only did he speak, he talked incessantly, relating every detail of situations or episodes that concerned him. Daniel worked alone because when he worked with others, he became so involved in explaining his concerns that he totally ignored his work tasks. Cognitively, Daniel is capable of much more than he is doing, but a way of harnessing his intelligence into work consistent with his capabilities had not yet been found. Community work positions are being developed for some of the adults in the programs. Whether Daniel will be one of them is questionable.

A good-looking man of about forty entered the shop and delivered something to the agency director. I was not sure whether he was a man with autism or a staff member. He quietly beckoned me to his side. "I'm very interested," he said in a soft voice, "in knowing whether you were born in Manhattan." After I answered affirmatively, he continued. "What hospital were you born in?" I gave its name. "What was the date of your birth? I'm just interested," he stated, trying to assure me that he meant no harm by this question. At this point I was rescued by my guide. "It's not appropriate to ask people that question when you've just met them," my interrogator was told.

Another man started to talk to my guide about his daily trips to the shop. He traveled independently by train and bus from another part of the city. With his long hair, laborer-type work clothes, and sturdy physique, he looked less like an easy mark for muggers than most people in this city. But his voice did not match his appearance. It would frighten off no one. Its high pitch was unexpected and had almost a whining quality. The words emerged slowly. This man had been expelled from several previous programs because of periodic aggressive episodes. Here, he had worked out a way to avoid them. Jim could now recognize when he was losing control, announce that he was leaving, and depart. He was becoming much better at self-management.

There was also the man I didn't see because he was no longer at the group home. What I saw instead were the plastered walls of what had been his room. He had punched big holes through two of the walls. Now he was the client of another agency, one that took the adults with whom other agencies could not cope. That man too could communicate.

A monthly meeting of a local chapter of the Autism Society of America featured a pianist. In fact, the meeting was primarily a concert, and the concert artist was a young man with autism. It is the evening of the meeting. We are told that he will play two pieces by Debussy and two other classical pieces. No music is in sight, but none is needed. He appears to have perfect concentration and plays with a high level of skill. Having completed this part of his program, he bows, smiles, and takes a seat in the audience. His mother says something to him, following which he returns to the piano and announces, "The pop stuff will be now." He begins with a selection from the Broadway show *Cats* and then continues without interruption through a long medley of show tunes, giving the impression that he could continue indefinitely. He seems very pleased with the enthusiastic response of the audience, even though only about twenty people are present, and several of them are family members or friends.

The pianist's mother then relates some of the details of his development, including his multiple tantrums each day during early childhood; his echolalic and then rote speech; his inability to eat solid food until age seven; the many schools he attended as his parents continued to search for better help; and his ability to play Mozart concertos before he was five, although he could not read music and had not yet received any formal instruction. It was not until his junior high school years that this special ability began to help him gain social success, as he became the star of the school orchestra even though he was in a special education class. His mother is obviously proud of him and proud of her own perseverance and determination in fighting against his autism. She summarizes his accomplishments: he drives a car, lives in his own apartment, works professionally as a pianist, has a pet, and has friends.

Then there is some time for questions. Would he care to tell us when language and people started to make sense to him? I asked the pianist. His father, sitting next to him, appears to be helping him with the question. Then the pianist stands up and responds: "My music and language came to me a long time ago, and there's no limit." Afterward, his mother adds: "He's still learning; there are still gaps." Yet the pianist has friends, apparently good ones. Some are there at his concert. His face lights up when he goes to greet them, and they regard him with obvious warmth. He lives independently and he works at what he loves. Recovered from autism? Not completely. But many would envy his life.

And let's take another look at Jessy Park. She is now known as an accomplished artist and sells her art work easily. One of her pieces sits on my office desk. It is Jessy's unique version of the Flatiron Building in Manhattan. She has made many paintings of this building. Lavender and pink are the colors that dominate the one I have, and the minute building blocks of this edifice are presented in detail. I have looked at the actual Flatiron Building in Manhattan numerous times over the years. What I saw was just a building, unusual in its shape but otherwise very ordinary. What Jessy Park saw and has shown me is a glorious work of art construed from her special way of perceiving the world around her, the "zillions of sensory details" of raw visual information that neurotypicals cannot access but that are accessible to some individuals with autism (Grandin and Johnson 2005, 67).

4 Families

Nobody can destroy a family quite like some autistic children . . .

(Hundley 1971, 87)

What is often stolen away by autism is the joy of being a child and the joy of being a parent—the "goodies" that come with having a child, is the way one parent put it. What is lost too is a sense of unlimited potential.

After I reread these statements and the rest of this chapter as I had written it in 1996 and 1997 for the first edition of *Targeting Autism*, I thought to myself, "No, this is not right!" This was the bleak world of autism for families then, in the 1970s, the 1980s, and the early 1990s. It's still the world of autism for some families, but not for most families anymore. I have to present all versions of the picture as they appear today, both the bleakness that still exists for many families and the more promising vistas unfolding for many others.

Why are the vistas for many families less somber today? Was it the inclusion of Asperger syndrome as one component of autism spectrum disorders? To some extent, this may be true, but that is not the whole explanation. Other factors have also come into play—greater awareness, earlier intervention, better intervention, and more parent support groups and networks have all contributed to the brightening picture for most children on the spectrum and their families.

All families go through different stages as children arrive, grow up, and move out, and as parents grow older. Each stage brings new challenges and demands new accommodations. All families experience stresses, and many suffer rifts and dislocations. What's particularly different about families in which a child has autism is that their source of momentum, and the fulcrum on which family life turns, is the individual with autism.

Some families fracture from the tension; some grow closer. Some parents experience crisis followed by breakdown; others endure periodic crises and get through them somehow; and still others encounter crisis followed by growth. Siblings may be slotted into roles as secondary parents and teachers. Many are ambivalent about this incursion into their childhood and the scant attention their own needs receive; others become wed to providing such care and become professionals in this area. Whatever the choices family members make and the outcomes of those choices, autism becomes the central experience in their lives for many years, sometimes for a lifetime. "Why is this happening to me?" a father asks. His wife is repulsed by his version of grief.

> "Our words are about to escalate into a well-rehearsed argument about who is getting enough time to work, who should be making child care arrangements, who will drive Elijah to the medical lab for his next blood level check. . . . I'm tired of this marriage," I say across the room. "I'm tired of our history. I don't know *us* anymore." (Paradiz 2002, 30–31)

Families can revolve around autism in many ways. Time is one of them. All other interests, activities, and friends not connected to autism get shunted aside, first because of the frantic search for information and a cure, or at least a powerful treatment, and later because time is for implementing treatment strategies. Everything else recedes into the deep background.

Autism also becomes a focal point because of money. It takes lots of it to put comprehensive treatment programs into place. Money becomes an issue: How much of it will it take? Can we manage that? How? If we can't, what do we do next? Where or to whom do we turn for help?

Autism is the axis around which the family revolves. Jobs are sacrificed; opportunities for advancement are postponed or given up. Families live apart or uproot themselves altogether from their communities to get their autistic children into better treatment programs, to get them a better chance to be cured. Craig Schulze gave up his job to live in Boston with his autistic son, while his wife and daughter divided their time between Maryland and Massachusetts, because the Boston Higashi school appeared to be his son's best hope, and Jordan needed his family.

Autism may become the nerve center of the family, as when parents are afraid to have additional children lest those children also be autistic, or because it would be unfair to any children to come, or because they couldn't manage other children and their autistic child. Josh Greenfeld reported a conversation he had about his then four-year-old son Noah with Ivar Lovaas of the University of California, Los Angeles, who was supervising Noah's treatment:

> "You worry too much about Noah. You should worry more about your other boy. Or maybe you should have another child. In that way you would worry less. . . ." "But I have eleven children already. To have an autistic child," I said, quoting a Long Island mother of a child like Noah, "is to have ten children." (Greenfeld 1972, 157)

Other children in the family recognize that the child with autism has the spotlight. One sister wrote: "An autistic child in one's midst requires extraordinary compromise for every member of that youngster's family. We all adapt as best we can, but sometimes the penalty for our constant accommodation is considerable" (Zatlow 1982, 50).

Parents of autistic children assume a multitude of roles in addition to those played by parents of typical children. They are searchers in quest of cures, or at least effective treatments. They are advocates, fighting for the services and supports they believe will give their children a better chance for a good life. They are therapists and therapy coordinators. Some parents fill these roles better than others do, but all parents grapple with them.

One mother kept searching until she learned about Landau-Kleffner syndrome and found that her son could benefit from the treatment used for this disorder. Another mother searched until she learned about auditory integration training and found that it improved her daughter's functioning. These were not established treatments for autism. Other parents have concluded that one of the better-researched approaches for children with autism, such as applied behavior analysis, is the best one for their child. It took time, energy, and dedication to engage in the searches that led to these conclusions.

Some parents, having searched and found what they believe is the most effective treatment currently available, are still driven. The best is not enough. What they seek is a cure, one they hope will help their own son or daughter as well as the children of others. These parents are the force behind many research efforts today. They establish research foundations, make donations to existing institutions for research on autism, prod the research community to focus more attention on autism. Autism continues to be the center of their lives.

Parents are the primary advocates for expanded services to autistic children, adolescents, and adults—their own and the children of others. The fifty-thousand-member Autism Society of America was founded by parents and is still a parent-driven organization. So too are Cure Autism Now (CAN) and many more. Grandparents are playing a significant role as well. The major functions of most of these groups are advocacy and raising funds for research. Autism is in the bones of the family members who make up such organizations.

Before the advent of federal laws mandating services to young children with disabilities, parents were often their sole teachers or their primary teachers. Many devised and implemented their own home treatment programs. Today parents more commonly act as co-teacher or co-therapist, treatment coordinator, and service monitor. Autism drives their lives.

In her book *Eating an Artichoke,* Echo Fling tells us about her role as a mother:

"You are his Annie Sullivan," said my husband. In a very real sense he's right. Throughout this child's life, I've been helping him interpret his environment. . . . I've been accused of sheltering my son from the challenges of life. I don't know of any mother of a child with AS who hasn't endured these onslaughts. (Fling 2000, 195)

At times it can become too much. Craig Schulze, unable to halt his son's deterioration and faced with making a dramatic sacrifice for his child, underwent a crisis and recognized that he had to heal himself. Lurline Morphett collapsed and briefly wound up in a mental hospital from years of tension accumulated in the process of raising her autistic son with very limited support.

Fantasies of getting rid of the autistic child may surface. One night Mary Callahan and her husband, driven to the edge by their young son's incessant crying but rejecting the idea of placing him in an institution, the only alternative they knew of at that time, had the following conversation:

"We could kill him." I was the first to say it.
"We could," Rich answered, looking down at his hands. "You could get something at work, couldn't you? An injection of something?"
"Yeah, but it would show up on autopsy. And if the drug didn't, the needle hole would."
We sat in silence a while longer.
"He could have an accident, like drowning in the bathtub or something," Rich said. . . .
"We'd go through life knowing we've killed our own son."
"We'd know we did it for him."
"We could never get a divorce," I said. We both laughed hysterically, unable to stop, even when we stopped thinking it was funny.
We talked for hours, able at last to admit our helplessness to each other. (Callahan 1987, 59)

Sometimes the autistic child may be at acute risk of abuse:

On the day in question he screeched in my ear just once too often. Something inside me snapped and I temporarily lost control. . . . I could not resist hurting him. I slapped him about the head, harder and harder, reveling in the release of my pent up emotions. I could feel them pulsing out of my hands with each blow.

When I eventually regained my composure I was horrified at what I had done. (Morphett 1986, 65)

Parents are not the only family members whose lives revolve around the autistic child. Autistic children are also the center of action in the lives of their sisters and brothers. Letters and other brief pieces by siblings of autistic individuals frequently appear in the *Advocate,* the newsletter of the Autism Society of America. Most, like the letter that follows, express love for the child with autism, with only passing reference to difficulties (as if it were wrong and bad to dwell on them).

> Dear *Advocate:*
> My brother is autistic. It is kind of hard living with him, but he is just like anyone else. I love him very much. I would rather have him as a brother than any other brother in the world. (Nickelsen 1996, 4)

Other statements, often from adult siblings, reveal more complex feelings and relationships:

> I always thought it was a trick. . . . This child who tore my hair, who scratched my hands and bit my arms, who broke all my things and scared my friends away. . . . I knew it was just a mean trick and I scratched back, fought back and made him listen to me, because, I said, "you're not special, you're playing a trick and I can see right through you." I made him play with me and I made him copy me. . . . That was many years ago. . . .
> I called him today because I love him so much and because I resented him and fought him and protected him for so many years. (Kiebala 1995, 10–11)

The boy who wrote the following letter was encouraged to express his feelings, and he did:

> Dear Doctor,
> My mom told me to write this letter because I can't come. It's about my sister Hannah. It's hard to live with Hannah, she's almost always mean to me. She bites, kicks, and hits me. . . . None of my friends want to come to my house because they think she's gonna do something to them. . . . Hannah is always bothering me so I got really mad at her. She

never gets in trouble. . . . I've gone to lots of shrinks, counselors, and doctors to try and learn about what to do about Hannah, but they never help much. Hannah always gets the attention because my mom is always dealing with Hannah. (Isaiah 1995, 7)

These three letters mirror common themes heard from siblings. Which type of response pattern is most typical of a sibling probably depends on a variety of factors, some of which parents can't control and some of which they can. An autistic sister or brother is easier to love and teach if she or he doesn't hurt you and doesn't break your cherished possessions. An autistic brother or sister may be easier to play with and teach if you have another brother or sister to help you do this. An autistic sibling may be easier to accept when you feel that your parents respect your rights too, when they understand why you're angry and give you some attention. Recognition of these response patterns doesn't make it easy for parents to change these situations. Lurline Morphett regretted not realizing how difficult life was for her nondisabled daughter, but she didn't know whether she could have made it better even if she had recognized her daughter's strain.

In the preface to her book *Siblings of Children with Autism*, Sandra Harris refers to the needfulness of the sisters and brothers of children with autism: "But when I listen to the voices of these young people in sibling support groups, or in individual conversations, I am struck by the urgency of their needs." Harris describes one mother who kept the needs of her nondisabled son in the picture while she coped with her autistic daughter:

My seven-year-old daughter who has autism broke one of her brother's favorite toys the other day. He was upset and wanted me to punish her. At first I thought it wouldn't do any good, but then I realized that even if she didn't learn anything, he would feel that I was standing up for him, and it would make him feel better. So, I sent her to her room. (Harris 1994, 97)

Why do some families who have a child with autism appear to fare better than others? For a multitude of reasons, some of them related to the nature of the child's characteristics and some existing independently.

Almost all parents of children with significant disabilities experience high levels of stress during some periods of their son's or daughter's development. Stress may come from grief, from exhaustion, from not seeing progress, from fear for the child's future, from anger over what is being sacrificed by other family members. Whatever the nature of the child's disability, some families do better than others because they cope better with stressful situations in general. Of course the characteristics of the child or adolescent with autism strongly affect the family's ability to cope. It is more difficult to cope effectively when you see your son injuring himself or hurting his sister or brother. It is harder when your child attacks you often and has prolonged tantrums. It is a formidable task to keep going in the face of periods of deterioration, when your child appears to be going backward or at best standing still in spite of all your efforts over years. Coping well becomes easier when the child with autism responds in some ways and begins to show signs of learning; when the child hurts himself or herself and others less often; and when these changes occur while the child is still young. A basically healthy family can then begin to recoup, tend to the needs of other family members, and retrieve the experience of enjoyment.

Families do better when they have strong support networks. Temple Grandin's mother credits her neighbors with helping both Temple and herself. Some families can count on friends, as another mother explains:

> One of my closest friends, Pam, a divorcee with four young children, phoned me one day to make a special request. She said in effect, "I insist that you bring Simon to my house at least once a week, that you continue to do this until he feels at home here. Then you must leave him with me for as long as you wish, and take a break for yourself." Overwhelmed to the point of tears I gratefully accepted her suggestion, and as it turned out Pam was one of the few people whom Simon was content to be with, and her youngest son, Jason, became his first playmate. (Morphett 1986, 66)

Other families receive crucial support from a grandparent who has a special relationship with the autistic child or youth and who provides the family with badly needed periods of respite. Judy Barron reports: "My mother . . . gave much of her attention to Sean. I drove him to her house after school several days a week, and the two of them spent afternoons together" (Barron and Barron 1992, 175).

When parents can't turn to family or friends, some find two other resources of support helpful. One of these is respite care services, the other parent networks. Respite care services allow parents to take a break, do something for themselves, or think about the needs of their other children. Many disability agencies provide respite care services, and they may be available at no cost to families. Unfortunately, such services, whether delivered in the family home or at an agency site, can turn out to be disastrous experiences when the respite care provider does not know the child and has not learned how to productively respond to his or her special needs. Valerie Paradiz, Elijah's mother, found someone in the community who was considered "odd" but was good for Elijah, and she was able to marshal the financial resources to pay this support person, Sharron. Sharron's unrecognized Asperger syndrome turned out to be both what enabled her to understand Elijah and what caused her to seem odd (Paradiz 2002).

Parents with children on the spectrum can often help each other:

> There were many days, especially in the beginning of treatment, that I thought I wouldn't make it through the day, much less through several months or years. I remember sitting alone in our home office one afternoon with tears streaming down my face. I'd had it with all the demands Ryan's therapy was putting on me, and I'd had my limit of people in my house. The very sound of my name made my skin crawl because if someone called my name, he needed something from me, and I had nothing left to give. As I sat there, the phone rang. It was another mother who has a child like Ryan. Although we didn't know each other well, we shared our pain and our stress. She had no answers on how to alleviate my pain, but she was, in fact, an answer. Just talking with her reminded me I wasn't the only one with these struggles. That empathetic conversation and that timely reminder made the stress more bearable, made me feel so much better. (Hamilton 2000, 309)

Many parents find that parent support groups are very useful. Sharing "disasters" and other experiences, listening to what worked and didn't work for other families, and finding out how other families cope give some parents a sense of connectedness that they find comforting. In 1996 the Beach Center on Families and Disabilities of the University of Kansas reported that there were over five hundred parent-to-parent support programs in the country, although these programs served parents of children with various disabilities. Some programs include one-to-one support, with parents of younger children being matched with experienced, trained parents of older children and adults. Support groups for siblings may also serve valuable functions, but they are less often available.

But some families fracture from the overwhelming stress. Elijah's parents faced not only autistic disorder in their beloved son but also seizures and the debilitating effects of the epilepsy medication needed to stop those seizures. The glue that had held Elijah's parents together, the mutual attraction and respect, had been weakened to the point that their bonds dissolved. Much later, after Elijah was well on his way to a future that looked brighter, his parents were able to become friends again.

The stories told by Liane Willey (1999, 2002) remind us that higher-functioning adults on the autism spectrum may also be parents. How does this affect their children? The children themselves may have a propensity toward autism because of the genes they inherit. In fact, Liane Willey has a daughter with Asperger syndrome. She refers to her other two daughters as "in-betweeners, those among us who carry two or three aspie tricks in their everyday bag" (2002, 19). "Shadow syndrome" is the name John Ratey and Catherine Johnson created for in-betweeners (1997).

What is it like to have a mother with Asperger syndrome?

> I know life with an Aspie mom can be very difficult on children. . . . I say the wrong thing at the worst time. . . . I make the most unusual requests and remarks, take things too literally, obsess on the words and actions of others and typically, I am the one who never quite gets the point. . . .
>
> I used to hope that I would be able to give my children my best side at all times. . . . It was never my intention to rely on them as much as I do. Things are often skewed in our family, turned so that the mom ends up relying on the children for their judgment and guidance. (Willey 1999, 104–5)

Arthur was thirty-five years old. His parents, aging and experiencing health problems, could no longer cope with having him at home. In addition, they were terrified of the possibility that Arthur's care would become his younger sister's responsibility. They had lived through Arthur being rejected by all the nursery schools within traveling distance when he was three and four and by the public schools at age five; his lack of speech until almost age six, by which time they had despaired of his ever speaking; his need for constant monitoring; and his suspensions from special programs. They had somehow dealt with all that and much more, but now, after Arthur had acquired some significant skills—he spoke fluently, dressed and groomed himself, prepared some simple meals, and engaged in a few activities in the neighborhood independently—his parents had almost reached the end of their endurance. Thirty-five years of fear about what might happen next had taken its toll. His constant repetitive questioning grated on them, as his need for sameness restricted their existence. When a new form of problem behavior appeared in their adult son, they couldn't cope with it.

Had Arthur's parents reached this point before the mid to late 1980s, the options available to them would have been quite limited; but it was the 1990s, and many more possibilities existed. Arthur's parents began to explore them. A short time later, when a family crisis occurred, respite care services were arranged for Arthur. This was the first time in thirty-five years that his parents had had a break from the continuous care of their autistic son. To their surprise and relief, no major catastrophe occurred during the time Arthur stayed in the home of a couple experienced in working with autistic adults. A year later, Arthur was living in a small group home and, after an initial difficult period of getting used to this change in his life, he was doing well. He had acquired his first friend and enjoyed some of the group's activities, while choosing not to participate in other activities. His sister visited him frequently because she chose to do so, and the two of them sometimes went to one of Arthur's favorite museums or to a new movie that he wanted to see.

And what of Arthur's parents? Having ordered their lives around Arthur's care for so long, they had to reorient themselves and figure out what to do with their newly found time. After a few weeks, they began to enjoy the quiet that had been missing from their home for so long. They now see Arthur on weekends, and he stays over at his family home on holidays and other special occasions when he chooses to do so. The tension has drained out of the family. As Arthur said over and over again in preparing himself for his move, "I'm a man now. It's time for me to move on." It was that time for his parents too.

We have been focusing on the stress that autism brings into families and the need for family support, but there is another side of this picture—love, devotion, pride, and a sense of purpose. It's easy to see in Wayne Gilpin, who compiled and published two books—*Laughing and Loving with Autism* and *More Laughing and Loving with Autism*—filled with anecdotes about his son and about the children of other parents whose lives had been enriched by their autistic children. It's there too in the many families in which no one has written a book or spoken at a conference.

No one asks for autism, just as no one asks for cerebral palsy or epilepsy or any other developmental disorder. It happens. We don't know how to prevent autism. We don't know how to cure it. Treatment outcomes vary greatly. Some families are able to create lives of satisfaction even though their sons and daughters have not lost their autism. Ruth Sullivan commented in an interview: "Joseph opened up a whole new world for me. . . . It's a cliché, I know, but it's been a wonderful life" (*Advocate* 1995, 35). Perhaps one day soon, when we know more about how to help all children with autism, most parents with sons and daughters who have autism will be able to respond to Ruth Sullivan's conclusion by saying "ditto."

PART TWO Treating Autism

5 We Have a Dream

I pass through my kitchen and notice a mishmash of photos taped to
the refrigerator door. They've been stuck up in the same place forever
it seems, and now the corners have yellowed and the tape is coming off.
These tattered prints . . . show pictures of beautiful waterfront homes
sitting on hillsides. . . . There was once a dream there, in those little
clippings. A fantasy that I could taste. . . . But now . . . I have a different
dream. I've forgotten perfect houses, furniture, linen, china, landscaped
gardens, the Martha Stewart lifestyle. . . . Something pushed magazine
dreams right out of my head.

It's the dream that my son will be happy, and will find a way to move
comfortably through this world.

When you have one big overpowering dream, a mother's dream, nothing
gets in the way of it. It has top priority at all times. It's as urgent as a
baby's cry. . . .

We reach, we strive, and it's all for one dream.

(Harland 2002, 127–29)

What is my dream? My dream is that somehow Noah slowly improves, and
everything else, all other dreams, are contingent upon that. But how will
he improve?

(Greenfeld 1972, 79)

One evening in April 1995, I caught a train to Westchester so that I could be at a conference on autism early the next morning. It was after 9 P. M. when I arrived at Rye, New York. Only one adult left the train, an African American woman carrying a large duffel bag and a boy of about five. When I entered the motel van that arrived a few minutes later, two well-dressed women were already in it. They were talking about their children's treatment programs of six to seven hours a day, whether to leave therapists alone with their children, and whether every treatment session should be videotaped for review by a senior therapist. How long did it take for your son to get used to the sessions? one mother asked. The other mother responded: He pretty much tantrummed for a month. Now he doesn't mind. They work for five minutes and then play for ten. And the therapists—they're in control. They know what the child can do. And the good thing is I can always get a consultation on the phone. It's worth the seventy dollars an hour.

Those two women and I were going to the same conference, "Behavioral Intervention in Autism: Stepping into the Future," as was the woman with the five-year-old who had been at the train station. So was a group of mothers from Staten Island whom I knew and now met at the motel. These wives of policemen, firemen, and teachers and, as I later learned, the African American mother were all struggling to provide for their autistic children the kinds of services that the Westchester families already had.

The performing arts center at the State University College at Purchase, with its high ceilings and bi-level design, is spacious, modern, and light. I walked about, listening to snatches of conversation while the continental breakfast was being served. "Did you hear about this new book on autism?" "Someone just lent it to me; I'll read it right after the conference." "Have you made any progress with his toileting? They should be able to get that by age four." "I was desperate. I called my mom and said, 'Mom, can you come for a month? I can't handle this.'"

The orchestra of the thirteen-hundred-seat auditorium was completely filled, as was the balcony as far back as I could see. Mostly women, mainly in their twenties or early to mid-thirties, with a few older women who might be grandmothers or professionals. Each of these people had paid a hundred dollars to be there that day, two hundred to attend the next day as well, and a total of three hundred if they had reserved a place at the dinner that evening. There was a sense of purpose, excitement, and great importance in the air.

The program began. *Foundation for Educating Children with Autism, Inc.,* appeared on the screen. The president of this Westchester sponsoring organization explained that it had been formed by parents in July 1994 to establish schools for young children with autism. The first school was to open in January 1996. The audience was interested but slightly impatient. They had come to see and hear the guru of this movement, O. Ivar Lovaas, professor of psychology at the University of California, Los Angeles.

Ivar Lovaas is of medium height, with gray hair and beard, and a slight accent left over from his Scandinavian background. He is both dramatic and informal. The cause of autism? "We don't have a clue. Probably a multiplicity of etiologies. Autism is a guess. . . . If we all focus on looking for the cause of autism we wind up in a blind alley. You can disagree on whether a child has autism, but if you look at behavior, you can plan intervention and measure effectiveness." Seemingly casually, he debunks other approaches: three or four times a year a special treatment for autism is invented; none of them work, he implies. Behavioral therapy doesn't assume a sudden breakthrough. It's a slow, stepwise process.

He illustrates and explains autistic behavior through videotapes, showing children at different points of the treatment process. We watch in fascination and something akin to horror the rocking, twirling, and pacing; the hand flapping and staring at fingers; the turning on and off of lights; the lining up of small objects; and the flicking of a stick. These are self-stimulating behaviors, we are told.

Then comes a more difficult and controversial subject—the treatment of self-abuse, referred to here as self-injurious behavior. The videotapes show children banging their heads against furniture, biting themselves, pulling out their hair, socking themselves. In the 1960s, Lovaas admits, he did use physical punishment to treat this behavior, and shock therapy was sometimes used. While it was effective in the short run, the suppression did not last. We don't use punishment now, he reports. If you ignore the self-injurious behavior it will go up initially, he tells us, but soon the rate will go down. We also reinforce the child for other behaviors every time there is a pause in the self-injurious behavior, he continues.

More videotape, this time Lovaas at the first session with a three-year-old girl. He seats her in a chair facing him, hooking his feet around the chair so that she can't escape. Then he stands her up. She screams but can't go anywhere. As soon as she sits down again he offers her food. She refuses it and begins to have a tantrum. He pulls her up and then verbally and physically directs her to sit. As soon as she is seated he gives her a glass of soda. She drinks it. Later he no longer has to physically guide her to sit. He pulls her up, tells her to sit, and she does. He substitutes social reinforcers for food. "G-o-o-o-o-o-o-d," he says, elongating that word immensely, and adding a hug. "Look at me," he adds. She looks and he reinforces her.

"You have to learn to be a bitch," he tells the parents in commenting on the videotaped session. "Say 'sit' in a loud voice; later you can lower it."

Lovaas directs the very full agenda for the rest of the day. He outlines the central features of the treatment program: forty to sixty hours a week plus informal teaching by parents for one to four years if the child recovers; otherwise, for the rest of life. Live videotapes are the high point of the day. Several children have been brought to the conference for demonstrations of the behavioral treatment developed by Lovaas. A therapist works with one child backstage while a simultaneous videotape of them is being shown on the very large stage screen.

The child, who is two and a half, puts blocks into a shape sorter and is reinforced with raisins. Being swung up in the air is used as another reinforcer, as is a few minutes to "go play." "Come here," the therapist says, and then "Good coming," when the child complies. "Sit" and "Good sitting" are coupled with a tiny piece of a Snickers bar. The therapist taps a block on the table when the toddler's attention wanders. This child, we are told, has been in treatment for close to forty hours a week for one month.

The other children are older and have been in treatment longer. A five-year-old is still having difficulty picking out some of the shapes the therapist names. He prompts her, pointing to the correct shape and saying its name. She watches the materials attentively. At one point she uses her right hand to hit her left one. A second therapist appears. "What's your name?" he asks her. She tells him her first name. "What's Momma's name?" She responds correctly. "What's your last name?" Correct again. We are told that this child was in therapy for six months before she said her first name. A year later her vocabulary consists of about 150 words, but she still expresses herself with nonspeech sounds when she is under stress.

Another child is shown reading word cards, writing letters, and writing her name. Her reinforcers are hugs, high fives, "Good girl," and a sense of accomplishment. "I did it," she says with obvious pride, after she wrote a letter the therapist named. "She's on her way to recovery," Lovaas comments.

Tumultuous applause is the response of the audience at the end of the day. This is what they came for—to hear the person who has provided them with hope, who has shown them a way. He has also uttered that word they pray for every day: recovery. This is the dream that brought them here from Kansas and Vermont and Vancouver, the dream of their children having what we think of as a real life. It was what made them clap and cry and then leave exhilarated, with new hope, renewed confidence, and a sense of determination.

What was happening here? Had Ivar Lovaas found the key to recovery from this terrifying disorder? How had he come to be viewed as a savior by so many families? And why then, when he had been doing and reporting on behavioral treatment for many years? Is recovery from autism really possible?

To answer the "how" and "why now" parts of this enigma, we have to turn to Catherine Maurice. In 1993 her book *Let Me Hear Your Voice* was published, and her two autistic children were its subject. Within a few months, through an article in a popular magazine and word of mouth among parents, her book became almost a cult item—the proof and the protocol for recovery. And Catherine Maurice credited Ivar Lovaas with the rescue of her children. It was his work, she wrote, that charted a path to the journey home.

Anne-Marie was the second child of Catherine Maurice and her husband, Marc. Like her older brother, Anne-Marie seemed perfectly normal at first, although somewhat somber and a bit too content with solitary play. Her parents thought of her as their shy and sensitive child. Still, she would lift her arms to be picked up as she called out for her daddy, laughing when he kissed her and tickled her. She would also seek out her mother and gaze at her lovingly. At eighteen months Anne-Marie fell silent. Gone was her "hi" and "bye" and approximation of "I love you." A few months later the diagnosis of autism was confirmed. And then, when their third child was little more than eighteen months old, it happened again.

Catherine Maurice is not your typical parent. She has a PhD, and she writes movingly and convincingly. Her description of initial joy, followed by glints of concern, and then full-blown anxiety about signs that could not be ignored made parents feel as if they were reliving their own experiences. So when she communicated her conclusion that the Lovaas approach was the only one that offered a chance of recovery, that she had used it in spite of her initial revulsion at some aspects of this method, and that this approach had saved her children, other parents listened.

The dinner speaker at the Westchester conference on behavioral intervention in autism was Catherine Maurice. She is a slim, rather attractive, dark-haired woman who spoke in a soft and tenuous voice. Both her children had completely recovered, she told the six hundred people who had been lucky enough to get reservations for the dinner. An evaluation confirmed this. Her daughter was doing well in a third grade class, and her son was in the first grade. "For many parents my children represent hope," she told her audience. Yet she also mentioned her "very fragile sense of security about my children."

Stories of individual children or even two of them, case studies if you will, are of great value, but they can also be misleading. What were the critical variables that allowed and enabled Catherine Maurice's children to recover? We don't really know. Would the same approach lead to the same outcomes with different children, with most children who have autism? Are many parents who try to replicate Catherine Maurice's methods going to be disappointed with the outcomes for their children? Undoubtedly. Should they be discouraged? Should professionals advise them not to expect or hope for this outcome? No. At the Westchester conference on autism I commented to a nurse from Canada on the likelihood that many of the parents there were going to be very disappointed when their children didn't recover. That's not true, she responded. "We've already been so hurt that we will accept this. I have two autistic children," she continued, "one retarded and one not retarded. Even if my retarded son doesn't recover, at least I'll know that I've given him the best possible chance I could." Is this mother right? I asked myself. I was impressed but not totally convinced, and Lovaas left me uncomfortable, uneasy.

I went back to New York City with the African American woman and her five-year-old son who had arrived on the same train as I had. They were the only black people I saw at the conference. We had begun talking at the dinner table the previous night. The presence of her strikingly beautiful young son had brought her many interested listeners. Coming to this conference had been a financial strain, she told me, but she would do anything to help her son. How could he survive the way he was? In Brooklyn? In their neighborhood?

I asked her about her son's schooling. He had been in a special preschool program for two years, she told me, but it hadn't helped. This year, in a public school class for children with autism, he had gotten worse. "He has an aide assigned to him now because he had started biting," she explained. She had tried to get her son into a class in his school where they did some behavioral training. It was a special program that parents had to volunteer for, but she was told there was no more room. "Does he speak at all?" I asked, as I had not heard a sound come from this child, who hardly left her arms. "He can talk," she replied. "Sometimes he says something to me, but not so often. Sometimes I work with him at home and he talks." She was very glad she had come to the conference, this mother told me. She had talked to many people who had promised her help.

Five months later I tried to contact that mother to find out whether any of the promised help had materialized and to ask how her son was doing. After several tries I reached someone who identified herself as the child's sitter. The boy was in the same school program as last year and no help had arrived, she told me after I explained why I was calling; but he was doing a little better now. His mother would call me back the next day, she promised. That call never came. Desperate parents have no time for people who have no real help to offer their child. This mother had the same dream for her child as did the mothers from Westchester and those from Staten Island. What was different were the resources she could marshal in the struggle to achieve that dream.

TODAY AND YESTERDAY

Hope and expectations have a way of winding down with time, when outcomes don't match dreams. The father of a recently diagnosed two-year-old attended a meeting of a local chapter of the Autism Society of America. He will not go there again, he told his family. Those people accept their children's autism. He will never accept autism. He will fight it until his son recovers. He will never stop fighting it.

Yet forty years ago this national organization was founded by a group of fighters. Their dream too was to defeat autism, in their own children and in the children of others. The organizing meeting took place in Teaneck, New Jersey, in November 1965. About sixty people were present. "We fell on each other," recalls Ruth Sullivan, one of the parents present. "It was heady. For the first time we had hope. . . . It was the most electrifying meeting I have ever been at in my life" (Warren 1984, 102).

In 1969 the fledgling organization had its first annual conference. That was also an exciting and exhilarating meeting with impressive people, including parents who went on to develop programs, serve as consultants, and write books about their personal experiences with autism. Glimmers of current issues or preludes to them pervaded that conference, along with goals now achieved. Ivar Lovaas was the luncheon speaker at the second conference, in 1970, his subject the "Strengths and Weaknesses of Operant Conditioning Techniques for the Treatment of Autism." His message, however, was quite different then: "The program does not turn out normal children, and should a child become normal as we treat him, then that no doubt, is based on the fact that he had a lot going for him when he first started treatment" (Park 1971, 39).

Recovery was not the theme of that conference over thirty years ago, but the possibility of a life of near-normal functioning was. Parents spoke with both pride and sadness of the achievements and continuing limitations of their adult children, still odd men out, still struggling to understand and be accepted in the social world.

Now let's fast-forward to 1995 again, this time to July and Greensboro, North Carolina. It is the 1995 national conference of the Autism Society of America. The electricity of the organizing meeting thirty years earlier is gone. Missing also is the fervor of the Westchester meeting that had taken place three months earlier. Lovaas is not on the program; nor was he on the program in 1994. There is little talk of recovery here. Improvement, programs, strategies, support for families, and recognition of adults with near-normal functioning appear to be the themes.

One of the general sessions is a panel report from an autism research symposium sponsored by the National Institutes of Health. A member of the audience asks a question about recovery. A distinguished psychiatrist on the panel replies that in his contact with over eight hundred individuals with autism he has never seen a person who has recovered. What he has seen is symptom remission with near-normal functioning.

This conference does not celebrate recovery or use it as a goal. Too many parents in this organization have been forced to give up this dream. There is Craig Schulze, presenter on a parent panel, the author of *When Snow Turns to Rain,* the story of his son's deterioration and his unsuccessful attempts to reverse it. And Connie Post, also on that panel and the author of two books of poetry about her autistic son, who was placed in a residential center at age six because the family was disintegrating under the barrage of his attacks on his mother and himself. And Clara Claiborne Park, a third panelist, author of *The Siege,* a book about the childhood of her autistic daughter Jessy, whom no miracle had transformed. You wouldn't have to observe Jessy for more than five minutes to know she's autistic, Clara Park stated at an earlier session. Recovery, when it is mentioned here at all, is referred to quietly.

The questions in my mind after experiencing the contrast of these two 1995 conferences were whether the still obviously autistic sons and daughters of many participants at the North Carolina conference would have been different, closer to normal, or recovered if they had been treated with Lovaas's behavioral program when they were young and whether most of the children of parents at the Westchester conference would still be obviously autistic fifteen or twenty years later. Had we been shown a way to rescue substantial numbers of children from the devastating effects of autism? Or were the two conferences highlighting different points in the life cycle of individuals with autism and their families?

We have some answers to those questions today. The dreams of some parents have been fulfilled, and the dreams of others almost met; but there still continue to be dreams that fade badly or die under the barrage of disappointed hopes over the years.

6 Is ABA the Answer?

INTERVENTION APPROACHES

Behavior analysis has played a vital role in revolutionizing treatment and training in developmental disabilities . . . freeing individuals from many behavioral and adaptive barriers that had kept them dependent and devalued.

(Favell 2005, 24)

Autism can be an implacable foe, as anyone who has struggled against it knows. What makes the battle particularly grueling is that the contours of this foe are shadowy; it takes on different shapes with different children and within the same child at different ages. And this foe holds children in a vise-like grip. To wage a successful battle against such an adversary takes fierce determination, and for many children the struggle has no end. Moreover, the battle cannot be waged by professionals alone or parents alone. It takes the combined efforts of a dedicated family, skilled professionals, and a child who (eventually) demonstrates the will and means to fight. The mother of the cum laude university graduate referred to in chapter 2 recalled: "I thought of my son as the count of Monte Cristo, slowly tunneling his way out of autism."

WHAT ARE THE MAJOR APPROACHES CURRENTLY IN USE, AND WHAT DO WE KNOW ABOUT THEM?

There is no currently available treatment for autism that will cure all children or even bring all children with autism to near-normal functioning. There is instead a history of supposed "breakthroughs" or "miraculous treatments" that turn out to significantly help only a small proportion of children with autism. Because of Catherine Maurice's story about her recovered children, many parents acted as if the Lovaas applied behavior analysis (ABA) approach used with those two children had almost miraculous therapeutic power. The real picture is somewhat different.

What excited large numbers of parents in 1995 and made them view Lovaas as a savior were the outcomes he reported—almost half the children who were treated with his model at the UCLA clinic he headed were reported to have "recovered." (He later changed his language from "recovered" to "best outcomes.") Most later studies using an approach derived from that model did not achieve the same outcomes.

In recent years, behavioral programs have acquired primacy, and applied behavior analysis is today considered the treatment with the strongest foundation of supportive data from research. But ABA is not the unidimensional intervention approach it appeared to be in the mid 1990s, when parents viewed it as synonymous with what Ivar Lovaas was doing and preaching. Behavioral interventions, while they all share some core principles, come in different "flavors." Discrete trial teaching, which was the primary strategy in the Lovaas UCLA Young Autism Project model, is not the central strategy in other behavioral approaches; and some behavioral approaches look very different from the ABA model reported by Lovaas.

People prefer neat solutions to problems. When I teach the introductory course in special education at Hunter College, I try to help students see the complexity of many educational issues. One day, after a two-hour class session on the inclusion of children with disabilities in mainstream programs, a student raised her hand and asked: "Well, is inclusion good or bad?" My answer to that question was that there are more useful ways of thinking about this topic, such as, What are the potential benefits and pitfalls of this strategy? What can be done to increase the likelihood that inclusion will be a valuable experience? How do alternative strategies compare in terms of potential benefits and pitfalls? These are the kinds of questions that need to be part of our thinking about any proposed approach, whether for an individual child with autism or for children with autism in general. And, in the end, values play a significant role in selecting educational treatment approaches, particularly when no approach can promise the outcome that is the dream of all parents.

No single form of treatment known today will enable all or even most children with autism to achieve essentially normal functioning. In the future we may identify such a treatment. In the meantime educational treatment remains the most effective approach for most children, even though it is not the miraculous cure for which most parents long and is only moderately effective for many children.

Temple Grandin gives much of the credit for her good functioning to early school experiences:

> At age two and a half I was enrolled in a nursery school for speech-handicapped children. It was staffed by an older, experienced speech therapist and another teacher. Each child received one-to-one work with the therapist while the teacher worked with the other five children. The teachers there knew how much to intrude gently into my world to snap me out of my daydreams and make me pay attention. Too much intrusion would cause tantrums, but without intervention there would be no progress. . . . I would tune out, shut off my ears. (Grandin 1995, 96)

About three years later Temple Grandin began attending a small mainstream kindergarten class in an elementary school. Her early schooling had many elements that are generally considered optimal today. She began receiving services before age three. She was provided with one-to-one instruction in language. The teaching staff intruded into her autistic world and interrupted her stereotyped activities, but they did so gently. Having received intensive special education services before age five, Temple was able to participate in a mainstream educational program by kindergarten age. In addition to school services she had an excellent home-based program, thanks to the governess who kept Temple and her younger sister busy with games and art projects and taught them to skate, play ball, and jump rope, all the while enticing Temple into staying connected to the real world.

What do we know about educational treatment for young children with autism, and what questions or issues still exist? There is virtually no disagreement about the value of early educational intervention. Over thirty years of data collected by federally funded educational projects for children under age five with various developmental disabilities point to this conclusion, as do several studies of programs specifically designed for children with autism. Moreover, the National Research Council in its 2001 report, *Educating Children with Autism,* strongly endorsed the need for and value of early intervention.

Until recent years, tools for identifying children with autism below age three were either not available or not very useful. Today we have tools for screening and diagnosing children with autism early so that educational intervention can begin with toddlers, and research studies are beginning to point the way to even earlier identification. In addition, awareness of the need for early identification has increased substantially, and routine screening by physicians for autism spectrum disorders in children eighteen to twenty-four months old has been recommended by the American Academy of Neurology and the Child Neurology Society as well as the American Academy of Pediatrics. The M-CHAT, a brief questionnaire to be completed by a parent, is one screening tool developed recently for such surveillance. It can be administered during a standard pediatric visit and can identify children at risk of an autism spectrum disorder who should be referred for a comprehensive evaluation.

Many early intervention programs have been established since the mid 1990s, and all states participate in providing and funding early intervention services. These services commonly include speech/language therapy or applied behavior analysis or both. Occupational therapy is also often provided.

There is also widespread agreement that educational intervention needs to be intensive if it is to make a significant difference in the functioning of many children with autism. "Intensive" refers to the amount of time directly focused on the individual child's learning—the number of hours each day and each week of such intervention, and the duration of the intervention, whether weeks, months, or years. Lovaas found that ten hours a week of one-to-one behavioral intervention was not enough, while forty hours a week often was. Forty hours was what most parents of young children with autism wanted after they learned about the outcomes reported by Lovaas. Twenty-five to thirty hours is what many professionals believe may be essential in helping children with autism achieve as close to normal functioning as is possible through educational treatment during the early childhood years. The National Research Council recommended a minimum of twenty-five hours a week of systematically planned educational activities, twelve months a year.

However, many, probably most, young children with autism receive far fewer than twenty-five to thirty hours per week of instruction directly focused on their learning through intervention programs. Children may be at a preschool program site for twenty-five hours a week, but if a group approach is used most of the time, only a fraction of those hours may be specifically focused on the learning needs of an individual child; and most children under age three receive far fewer than twenty-five hours a week in early intervention services. In recognition of the need for more intensive intervention, early intervention systems are asking parents to participate more actively in the delivery of services through learning experiences in the home.

All intervention programs attempt to help the young child with autism become more responsive to his or her environment, particularly to the people in it, but it is here that educational intervention approaches begin to diverge. If we look at how different programs handle initial encounters with children, this point of divergence becomes clear. Some programs use rather forceful means of intruding into the child's autistic world, while others rely on a combination of enticement and gentle intrusion. Some begin by directing the child to imitate a standardized set of motor activities, rewarding imitation with something the child likes, often a potato chip or part of a cookie. Others start with an activity the child enjoys, such as riding on a swing or being tickled, but interrupt it to try to elicit some kind of communication from the child to ask for more. Still others begin by joining the child in his or her preferred activities and attempting to engage the child in interaction about them.

In programs based on or derived from the Lovaas Young Autism Project model, intrusion begins immediately. The initial program objectives usually call for getting the child to attend to the therapist ("Look at me"), follow simple directions ("Sit down; stand up"), and imitate actions modeled by the adult, such as dropping blocks in a bucket (Taylor and McDonough 1996). Directions are given in a loud voice. Physical guidance is used to ensure that the child follows the adult's directions, with food or other rewards used to reinforce the child's compliance. Some young children cry and seek to escape from their instructional sessions for many days after they are initiated into treatment programs. Catherine Maurice experienced this forcefulness as she watched her daughter being initiated into her behavioral program:

> As soon as Bridget placed Anne-Marie in the opposite chair the crying broke out in earnest. Anne-Marie tried to get out of the chair; Bridget kept placing her firmly back in. She collapsed on the floor; Bridget picked her up and put her back in the chair. She tried to put her hands in front of her face; Bridget took them down and held them in her lap.
>
> Anne-Marie was terribly fearful and distraught. She turned and looked directly at me, for the first time in weeks. Her mouth was trembling.
>
> I was cold and clammy with tension. Was this right? Was I doing the right thing? But I had wanted an assault. Hadn't I decided that we were going to "drag" Anne-Marie out of autism? (Maurice 1993, 87)

This starting point not only paves the way for later program objectives such as imitation of speech sounds but also establishes a pattern for child/therapist interactions: the adult directs, models, prompts, and reinforces; the child responds with imitation and compliance. In commenting on early intervention strategies, Temple Grandin remarked that while she was one of the autistic children who could be jolted into attention by her teachers, other children with autism—Donna Williams was one example—would withdraw or collapse altogether in the face of sharp intrusion into their autistic world.

In recent years behavioral programs have been modified to reduce the stress experienced by some young children at the beginning of treatment (Lovaas 2003). Most behavioral programs no longer insist on eye contact during this period or use physical prompting to achieve it. Lovaas has acknowledged that building eye contact is more difficult than he initially conceived and that pressing for it early in the treatment process may be counterproductive with some children. Loud voices are no longer common.

Most nonbehavioral approaches view forceful intrusion as counter-productive to the goal of motivating the child to want to communicate and interact with others. So, too, do some current behavioral models. Nonbehavioral programs that favor enticement of the child into more interaction usually begin quite differently. The adult usually takes his or her lead from the child's behavior, attempting to expand the child's inter-est in interacting. At the start of treatment the adult may match the child's actions or join in the child's activity focus. This matching of the child's actions horrifies some behaviorists who are intent on eliminating the autistic child's stereotyped behavior and eliciting compliance with adult directives. Yet mirroring of the child's behavior as a way of captur-ing attention and facilitating interaction is not without support from research or practice.

Mutual imitation is characteristic of the interactions of infants and their caregivers. Research with young autistic children by Geraldine Dawson and others has shown that when the adult imitates the child's behavior, the child displays more social responsiveness, for example, increased eye contact, touching, vocalizing, and toy exploration. Dawson speculated that allowing the child rather than the adult to lead the inter-action enabled the child to regulate the amount of stimulation received from the other person, thus avoiding painful overstimulation. Behavior-ists and others might ask why the normal process of mutual imitation that failed the autistic child in infancy should work now. Dawson rea-soned that this strategy might be effective if it was provided in mega-doses and was simplified for the child by the elimination of distracting environmental stimuli.

Stanley Greenspan (Greenspan and Wieder 1998, 1999) is probably the leading theorist in the area of developmental, relationship-based inter-vention with very young children. His followers include many psychologists, teachers, social workers, speech/language therapists, and occupational therapists involved in working with children from infancy through early childhood years and their families. Greenspan, too, believes in intrusion into the world of the child whom he refers to as having a "neurodevelopmental disorder of relating and communicating," a term roughly equivalent to autism spectrum disorder. But to Greenspan the intrusion must be congruent with the child's behavior and must focus on the child's affect. His intervention approach—the Developmental, Individual-Difference, Relationship-Based model (DIR), also referred to as Floortime—includes following the child's lead, joining in and expanding what the child is doing; but it also includes staging challenging problem-solving interactions designed to create new skills (Greenspan and Wieder 2005). The first goal of such intervention is shared attention and engagement. If a child is avoidant, Greenspan advocates being persistent in pursuit but playful.

Greenspan and his associates have worked with hundreds of young children with autism spectrum disorders using his intervention model. Parents are the major deliverers of in-home services, with professionals modeling, training, planning, and demonstrating strategies. School-based versions of DIR are also beginning to appear. In a review of the records of two hundred children whom he and Serena Wieder had followed for at least two years, Greenspan reported that 58 percent had good to outstanding outcomes, which included no longer scoring in the autistic range on the Childhood Autism Rating Scale (Greenspan and Wieder 1998). However, for multiple reasons, these data are not considered to reflect good research.

Barry Prizant, a communication disorders specialist who has extensive experience with young children on the autism spectrum, also uses a developmental approach and believes in enticing young children into interaction. He delineates a number of "Intervention Strategies to Entice Communication," which include the following:

> Place desired objects so that they are visible to the child but out of the child's reach or in containers that the child needs help opening.
> Engage the child in an activity that necessitates a utensil, then withhold the utensil or "sabotage" the function of the utensil.

Offer the child items that the child does not like or that the child does not need for an activity he or she is engaged in.

Set up a turn-taking routine for three or more turns until the child anticipates the steps and then violate a step in the routine. (Prizant and Wetherby 1989, 13)

Let's look at some illustrations of how the treatment of very young children with autism differs in programs with these different approaches. Melinda entered the Karen Horney Therapeutic Nursery at age three and a half. She had difficulties in relating, poor receptive language, and speech that was largely echolalic. She had areas of competence, too. She could recognize numbers, letters, and colors and could name some objects. Melinda was also hyperlexic. She could "read" (name) the words in children's books without understanding the meaning of what she was reading.

Melinda's teacher began the treatment program by trying to develop reciprocal play with her. The teacher and Melinda took turns blowing bubbles, playing peek-a-boo in front of a mirror, and throwing a ball back and forth. They worked on strengthening Melinda's relationship to her mother through visits to the parents' room during the school program, by using photographs of her mother in the classroom, and by making frequent references to "Mommy." The teachers drew pictures of Melinda at various activities, creating story books by adding written descriptions of what she was doing in each picture. They also put together books of photographs of Melinda and other people in her life. Staff used simple, functional language with her and tried to elicit the same from her. Melinda appeared to become more attached to her mother and more aware of herself. Her speech began to reflect her preferences, for example, "I want bike." "I want cracker." She also began to initiate dramatic play (Koplow et al. 1996). Melinda's program was consistent with a developmental approach like that of Greenspan or Prizant.

Nelson was not quite two, and he made no attempt to communicate. His mother had sought early intervention services because Nelson's four-year-old brother had autism, and Nelson had been diagnosed as having PDD-NOS. I watched this tiny boy and the young woman who had been his teacher for one month work within a behavioral format in a center-based class for toddlers. They sat facing each other on child-size chairs. Nelson's teacher was trying to get him to imitate her actions.

"Hands up," she said as she raised her arms. Nelson lifted his arms and was rewarded with a cheese doodle. Clapping hands was next, and another cheese doodle followed. Then the teacher blew soap bubbles toward Nelson, saying "bubble," "bubble," with an emphasis on the *b* sound, while Nelson watched. Some gentle tickling came next, and Nelson laughed out loud. "Look at me," the teacher said, holding a raisin in front of her face. It was then again time for hands up, but this time Nelson rejected the cheese doodle, and his teacher quickly substituted a toy piano designed for toddlers. Nelson cautiously pushed the keys. When bubble time arrived again Nelson went after a large one, broke it, and laughed.

The teacher changed activities. She pulled Nelson up from his chair and then told him to sit down. When he did this, the teacher gave him either a raisin or an opportunity to play briefly with a toy. After this pull up–sit down routine was repeated three times, Nelson began to cry. The teacher stopped, comforted Nelson briefly, and repeated the pull up–sit down exercise once more. Then it was time for a break, and after Nelson found that he couldn't open the room door, he did some jumping and ball throwing with assistance from his teacher.

What had Nelson learned? That if he imitated his teacher's actions and did what she told him to, he would get things he liked to eat and interesting toys to play with. He seemed to have grasped the idea of imitation and may have been in the process of learning to understand some simple verbal phrases. He also seemed to relate well to his teacher, allowing her to provide him with comforting and fun. This instructional session was a far cry from some of the harsh interactions that used to be common in behavioral programs. Nelson, however, made it easy to avoid harshness. He made no attempt to hurt anyone, displayed few stereotyped behaviors, and was compliant most of the time. Only when the teacher pursued mass trials, repeatedly directing Nelson to "sit down" after he had been pulled to a standing position, did Nelson appear to experience distress. Nelson's program was a modified, gentler version of a Lovaas-type ABA model.

The Language and Cognitive Development Center of Boston, founded by Arnold Miller, has been treating children with autism for over thirty years. Its treatment approach combines developmental and cognitive strategies in often inventive ways to entice the child to interact and become engaged. The focus of the treatment is on expanding the child's behavior and interactions with others. Jack, two and a half years old and diagnosed with autism, sat on his mother's lap at the beginning of treatment. He was handed pictures of animals one at a time every four or five seconds, before he could lose interest or throw the picture. But before receiving the next picture, Jack had to drop the picture in his hand into a nearby jar. Initially his mother helped him with this task. Next Jack and his mother moved to a table, where they sat across from each other. Jack's mother then sent the animal pictures to him in a toy truck that she rolled across the table. Now Jack had to insert the picture into a slot in the jar lid in order to get the next picture. A few sessions later, Jack had to send a picture by truck back to his mother. When she received a picture, she held it up and named all the parts of the animal. At a later point a toy barn with animal figures was introduced; human figures were added afterward. Through such a process Jack's interests, social interactions, and communication were expanded substantially within six months.

Each of the treatment approaches illustrated in these examples appeared to be effective with the particular child with whom it was used. Would the same approaches have been effective with other types of children—those who were older at the start of treatment, more severely impaired, more difficult to interest in any kind of interactive activity? Would they have been as effective if the three children had been switched around, with Jack going to the therapeutic nursery, Melinda to the behavioral program, and Nelson to the language and cognitive center? Perhaps not, although these are questions we cannot yet answer with any degree of certainty.

Children who started treatment at the Language and Cognitive Development Center before age three, as Jack did, had significantly better outcomes with this approach than did those who began treatment later, according to the center's directors. And while the center reported that 48 percent of the children it treats "have returned to their regular public schools able to mainstream in some or all of the classes," these data are referred to as providing only "a rough measure of the Center's effectiveness" (Miller and Eller-Miller 1989, 496).

It is also hard to judge to what extent Melinda's good progress was typical. Therapeutic nursery programs have become much less common, and when they report effectiveness data at all, the reports are usually presented as selective case studies. The curriculum used in therapeutic nurseries is generally rich, and harshness finds no place there. The traditional therapeutic nursery had as its foundation a combined developmental-psychodynamic approach highly consistent with Stanley Greenspan's DIR model. The key dynamic was nurturance—nurturing a sense of self and nurturing expression through engagement in play. While this approach may be wonderful for some children with PDD-NOS who can understand speech and have begun to communicate, it may not do well for more severely impaired autistic children. Some programs that keep the "therapeutic nursery" title now incorporate additional strategies, including behavioral programming, into their models.

In one therapeutic nursery I observed an autistic boy who was almost five. He was sitting in a sandbox filling a bucket and then pouring the sand out or letting it slip through his fingers, much as Temple Grandin used to do on the beach when she was very young. Another child sat no more than two feet away from him, but he appeared not to notice her. An assistant teacher tried to join his play, to expand it. The boy moved to another area of the room. He did allow the teacher to hold his hands as he jumped up and down on a mini-trampoline, and his smile confirmed that this was something he enjoyed; but what else was he getting out of this preschool experience? What kept going through my head as I watched him was that he would soon be five, had no system of communication, appeared to have little understanding of speech, largely avoided interaction, and engaged in stereotyped play activities. This is not an appropriate intervention program for this child, I kept thinking, and critically valuable time is being lost.

Applied behavior analysis is the educational treatment approach receiving the most attention today. What do we mean when we say that the approach used in a particular program is behavioral or that a program uses applied behavior analysis? A simplified explanation is that a behavioral treatment approach is based on two major principles of learning:

children will increasingly engage in behavior that is rewarded (reinforced); and behavior *not* reinforced will, perhaps after an intervening period, occur less and less frequently.

A behavioral approach to the treatment of children with autism is also associated with certain program components. *Discrete trial teaching* is a core strategy in the Lovaas Young Autism Project model and in many other behavioral programs for children with autism. This term refers to direct instruction that focuses on one specific bit of knowledge or skill at a time, with repeated practice (mass trials) on this task. Nelson's teacher was using discrete trial teaching when she repeatedly pulled him up from his chair and then directed him to "sit down." She would continue to repeat this process several times during the day over a period of perhaps weeks until Nelson demonstrated consistently that he responded correctly to the phrase "sit down."

The term "applied behavior analysis" also refers to a systematic process of observing and recording an individual's behavior and then using the information collected to shape instruction. ABA provides the "technology" or tools for intervention. And yet, in the end, effectiveness is to a significant extent determined by the knowledge, skills, and creativeness of the educators who collect, analyze, and use the data to design individual educational treatment strategies.

Behavioral programs for young children with autism generally use a one-to-one teaching format during their initial phase. The National Research Council endorses one-to-one or very small group instruction to meet individualized goals. Programs using such a teaching format are expensive, though in the long run they could prove to be economical by demonstrating a distinct advantage in enabling students with autism to enter mainstream educational programs later on in childhood. Currently, however, a one-to-one format is used sparingly in publicly funded school-based programs for children with autism, whether with preschoolers or with children five and over. What is seen much more frequently are classes with six or more students, one teacher, and a teaching assistant or sometimes two assistants.

When a Lovaas-type behavioral program is working as designed, it goes something like this: as soon as autism is recognized an intensive (forty hours a week or close to it) one-to-one program is instituted in the home. Discrete trial teaching is the major instructional strategy until the child has made considerable progress, and it remains the major strategy for new types of learning. The treatment program usually lasts three years, with imitation and following simple directions the major focuses during the first year, communication and interactive play the second year, and socialization and adjustment to school and community settings the third year. When the child demonstrates that he or she can learn from observation, has some rudimentary communication skills, and does not frequently exhibit tantrums, aggression, or self-injurious behavior, he or she begins to attend a preschool program for typical children on a part-time basis, accompanied by a teaching assistant who is associated with the child's in-home program. The child continues to have one-to-one instructional sessions at home. By age five or six, the child begins attending a kindergarten class with children who are either age peers or a year younger. Other types of placements are considered for children who appear likely to need ongoing and substantive special education services.

Lovaas's Young Autism Project outcome report was bombarded with criticism during the 1990s. The most persistent and forceful criticism focused on his claim that 47 percent of the children served in the Young Autism Project, nine out of nineteen, had "recovered" or had "best outcomes" (Lovaas 1987). Critics called this claim highly misleading, and it was. For one thing, Lovaas had excluded from the study children with autism who had extremely low IQs or who were between forty and forty-six months old but had no speech—in other words, children who were very likely to have poor outcomes. Parents of children who wouldn't have been considered for the project because they didn't meet the criteria expected their children to have an almost even chance of achieving normal functioning or something very close to it. They didn't. A later analysis of gains made by children with initial IQs below 35 who had received intensive services using the Lovaas UCLA model showed only modest improvement. On follow-up, the mean IQ of this group of children was 36, and only one child's adaptive behavior had improved, although ten of the eleven children had acquired some communicative speech (Smith et al. 1997).

Whether children were referred to as "recovered" or as having achieved a "best outcome," and even with the issue of excluding children with very low IQs set aside, serious questions were raised about the outcome data reported by Lovaas. One of the nine children who made up the "best outcome" group was later moved into special education, thus reducing the percentage of successful outcomes from 47 percent to 42 percent (although another child was later moved from special education into the mainstream and met the criteria used by Lovaas for "best outcome"). Moreover, the second follow-up study of this group of students, which was to have traced their progress into adulthood, was not completed, although Lovaas reported verbally that the six of the nine individuals evaluated as part of this follow-up still met the criteria for "best outcome."

In the 1990s many agencies and parents attempted to implement intervention programs based on the Young Autism Project. The Lovaas UCLA clinic offered training to parents via workshops and follow-up support by clinic staff. However, few parent-managed programs achieved anything close to the outcomes reported by Lovaas. Nor have most agency-run programs derived from the Young Autism Project model achieved "best outcomes" comparable to those claimed by Lovaas.

Some time ago, I visited a school for children with autism that used a model based on the Young Autism Project and aimed at recovery. The director was well trained and highly regarded. How are the preschool children doing after a few years? I asked her. We don't have the same recovery rate as Lovaas, she replied. A couple of our former preschoolers are now in inclusion programs, she told me, but for most of our preschoolers, placement in a less restrictive special education class is a more realistic goal. The children who make very modest gains stay here.

Another criticism often directed against behavioral programs similar to the Young Autism Project model is that they produce rote or nonfunctional learning, that children learn to give certain responses during formal instructional sessions in the classroom but don't apply this learning in appropriate situations unless they are prompted to do so. Thus, a child may have learned to say "I want juice" during work sessions, but doesn't use this language during lunch at school or at other times at home even if he or she likes and wants juice. In fact, such criticism was often justified in past years, but it is much less often justified today. Good behavioral programs today include teaching in a variety of functional situations, for example, practicing use of language for requesting foods within the context of lunch, and practicing words about clothing in the context of a child putting on a hat and coat to go home. Such functional teaching is not used to replace formal instructional sessions using a discrete trial format, but rather to complement and supplement it to promote generalization.

In a similar vein, programs derived from the Young Autism Project model have been criticized for focusing on reactive behavior, that is, teaching children to respond to adult directives and questions, to the detriment of spontaneity, initiative, and decision making. This criticism had considerable merit in the past and still does to some extent, although some behavioral programs have modified their instructional planning to include opportunities for children to choose, decide, lead, and initiate. Still, this is an area in which there is considerable room for more improvement.

A parent wrote to the editor of a journal with the following question:

> My 19-year-old son has autism and moderate mental retardation. He has had a pretty good education and had a lot of discrete trial instruction as a boy. . . . But, my son almost never asks for anything. I know he wants something because he will point or try to reach for things he wants. . . . If I ask him what he wants he will name the item. . . . He has a very good vocabulary and can name just about every item he might want. What can I do to make him less passive?

The associate editor responded:

> It sounds like your son had a great deal of discrete trial teaching (DTT) that was highly useful to him, but not enough early teaching in how to initiate and make requests. Those of us who come from an Applied Behavior Analysis background tended to rely very heavily on DTT in years past, but more recently have been placing a greater focus on more naturalistic teaching and the encouragement of spontaneity. (Harris 2005)

The most severe criticisms leveled against behavioral programs are judgments of such approaches as they were implemented in the past. First, there is the association between behavioral programs and punishment. Yes, behavioral programs often used "aversives" in their treatment during the 1970s and 1980s; and there remained a sharpness or harshness in these programs throughout most of the 1990s that dismayed many parents and professionals, including me. Some school programs used restraint holds with young children whenever the students exhibited aggression of any type. This practice was built into students' individualized education programs with parental permission and sometimes became a major intervention strategy.

I once watched a "therapist" use a loud voice to address a five-year-old boy, with her face only a few inches from his. It was a strategy she had been taught for getting his attention. Stereotyped actions like hand flapping often drew a loud "no." Such responses were derived, to a considerable extent, from the strong focus on the elimination of undesirable behavior that was present in many behavioral programs and from the blessing Lovaas initially gave to harsh intrusion and other kinds of tough treatment. Such harshness of response to children's behavior has declined significantly since the mid 1990s. In recent years, I have seen and heard a lot more hugging, kissing, tickling, swinging, praising, ignoring, and tolerating in most behavioral programs I visited than I did sharpness.

And finally there are the children who stay in Lovaas-type behavioral programs for long periods of time as the gap between themselves and typically developing children grows wider and wider. What parents and professionals often forget is that more than half of the children treated in the Young Autism Project study did not achieve anything approaching normal functioning, and some made only modest progress although they stayed in the treatment program for several years. One child was kept in treatment until his early teens, receiving more than fifteen thousand hours of therapy without acquiring much functional speech, and in the end his IQ had declined (Lovaas and Buch 1997, 82).

I again watched a videotape of five boys from the Lovaas Young Autism Project, three of whom were considered "recovered," one considered to have made substantial progress, and one to have made only modest progress. Fourteen-year-old Chris, the example of modest progress, functioned better than many autistic adolescents with severe mental retardation. Although he was in a class for retarded and autistic students, had an IQ of about 30, and used signs because of his limited speech, we see him eating appropriately at the table with his mother and brother and shooting baskets in the family yard. No person and no approach produces good outcomes with all children who have autism, even when intervention begins at a young age, as it did with Chris. Chris and his mother still had structured sessions focused on such tasks as naming objects from pictures. When Chris turned away during this session, his mother told him sharply, "Look." Whenever his face moved into a tic-like grimace, she shouted, "No faces!" For two years she had been teaching him to set their dining room table so that when he reached age twenty he might be able to work as a busboy. I wanted to tell this mother, very gently, that there are better ways to help her son to adulthood, that it was time to move on and probably had been for quite a while. How many times had she shouted "No faces!" at her son? I wondered.

Although many small studies indicated that programs based on the Young Autism Model did not achieve outcomes as good as those reported by Lovaas and his associates, nonetheless this approach appears to have a distinct advantage over programs with so-called eclectic approaches that provide the same number of hours a week of intervention (Howard et al. 2005). The "eclectic" program model in the study that reported this finding combined a system known as TEACCH (Treatment and Education of Autistic and Related Communication-Handicapped Children), some ABA, and sensory integration training. It is interesting to note that a small recent study found TEACCH superior to an eclectic approach (Mesibov, Shea, and Schopler 2004). What may be operating here is that programs without a clearly defined and cohesive approach do not provide the consistent and skilled implementation found in clearly delineated models.

A multisite replication of the Young Autism Project, funded by the National Institute of Mental Health, has been in progress for about ten years, and outcome data from these replication sites have been awaited eagerly. Lovaas has long claimed that other programs using this model have not achieved the same outcomes as originally reported because they were not faithfully replicating critical aspects of the model, especially intensity, staff training, and skill levels. Apparently, researchers encountered many problems in carrying out this study, including a large number of program sites that withdrew or were dropped. There were also delays in reporting data because the planned two years of treatment on which outcome data were to depend turned out to be insufficient for achieving outcomes like those originally reported by Lovaas. Furthermore, substantive changes in procedures were incorporated into the model at the replication sites, including reducing the number of consecutive practice trials from ten in a row to only two or three and incorporating more play into the treatment sessions. Eleven sites, six of them in other countries, completed the study, and data began to appear at the end of 2005. At one site, the original Lovaas outcomes were achieved, but only after four years rather than two (Sallows and Graupner 2005). Reports from other replication sites are still being awaited.

Robert Koegel was involved in implementing the Lovaas Young Autism Project at UCLA in the 1970s and 1980s. Since then he and his wife, Lynn Koegel, who together direct the Koegel Autism Research Center at the University of California, Santa Barbara, have evolved their own "brand" of behavioral intervention. The Koegels focus on pivotal behaviors such as motivation, responsivity to multiple cues, self-initiations, self-management, and empathy (Koegel and Koegel 2005; Koegel and LaZebnik 2004).

In an April 1997 conference presentation Robert Koegel reported that his own thinking about intervention had been challenged by the lack of happiness apparent in the children in the Young Autism Project even when they were making progress. He wanted children to want to learn to communicate and interact. In the attempt to make this happen, different objectives and methods came to the fore. In a Lovaas-type model, motivational considerations were generally limited to identifying good reinforcers for a particular child. In the newer model advocated by the Koegels, the focus on motivation as a pivotal behavior brings into the process the child's preference or choice of instructional materials (stimulus materials, in behavioral terms), as well as teaching in the context of play and functional activities and the use of natural reinforcers.

With this approach, the young child who points to a toy car and then looks at the teacher gets the opportunity to play with the car rather than receiving a bit of food or some tickling. Instead of teaching colors by presenting paper circles or triangles of different colors, the teacher might hold out a handful of M & M candies. If the child takes an orange one, the teacher might say: "Orange. Take orange. What color is this? Orange." When all the orange M & M candies are gone, the same procedure can be repeated with the next color the child chooses, and this procedure can also be carried out with other kinds of items the child likes. The reinforcement for the child was getting to eat the M & M or play with the requested toy—natural reinforcement that is very different from giving a Frito to a child who names the color of a circle correctly. Fritos might be used, according to Robert Koegel, to teach a child to open a lunch box when it contains this snack. Pivotal Response Treatment does not use mass trials of adult-selected tasks unrelated to the child's likes and activities. Tasks are varied to sustain the child's interest, and any attempt by the child to respond is reinforced.

Some time ago, I visited a preschool with a Lovaas-type behavioral program. One little girl would not stay with her teacher during the formal discrete trial instructional period. She kept leaving her seat and wandering around the room, listless, not appearing interested in anything in particular. "What's wrong with her today?" one of the other teachers asked. "She has no motivation," replied the girl's teacher. "All the [potato] chips are gone." Had Robert Koegel been there, he might well have commented: That's how we operated in the old days, and that's what needed to be changed.

Pivotal Response Treatment is an approach that has garnered much attention recently. It is supported by considerable research data and is consistent with the latest trends in intervention thinking. It addresses the following conundrum described by a mother of a child with severe autism: "We can teach her one new skill, or five, or ten. . . . But there are hundreds of such skills inherent in the condition of a normal eight-year-old" (Park 1982, 263). This mother's lament highlights another important dilemma in educating children with autism. Autistic children don't learn much in the natural course of childhood activities and don't generalize from one situation to another unless their instructional programs give them extensive practice in doing so. Even with such practice, generalization is not assured. How then can we possibly teach a child with autism all he or she needs to know to behave normally and acquire age-appropriate skills?

The answer is that we can't—if we try to teach every skill individually. The combination of the child's difficulty in generalizing and the use of teaching approaches that focus on a series of single skills accounts for some of the inappropriate behavior and misconceptions seen in older children and adolescents with autism. Robert Koegel and Lynn Koegel have attempted to deal with this problem by focusing on what they call "pivotal behaviors"—behaviors that are likely to affect many areas of functioning. In doing so, they are incorporating into an applied behavior analysis framework some of the more naturalistic teaching techniques common in preschool programs that have a developmental framework.

In more naturalistic approaches such as Pivotal Response Treatment, the child has more choice and more control. If a child is grumbling because he or she doesn't want to do something, the teacher says, "If you don't want to do it, say so." And if the child does this, he or she can change activities—again, natural reinforcement. Much disruptive behavior disappears with this approach.

The pivotal behavior of responsivity to multiple cues is important because children with autism may identify complex objects or situations on the basis of only one or two marginal cues. Victor, a nine-year-old boy with autism, did not recognize the psychologist whom he had known for four years when she came into my classroom one day without her cane. Although he had always gone to her office willingly on earlier occasions, on that day he refused to go with her, saying he didn't know her. Only after another student retrieved the psychologist's cane from her office did Victor recognize her. He then readily agreed to leave with her. Children with autism often have overselective attention.

Traditional behavioral programs rely heavily on an adult's control of undesirable behavior by such means as extinction—the removal of reinforcers, including attention. Self-management as a pivotal behavior involves teaching the child skills such as identifying appropriate behavior in different types of situations and monitoring his or her own behavior for such appropriateness. The process of self-monitoring shifts the locus of control to the child, who then learns to function more independently.

Victor used to find it very hard to wait for my attention without becoming upset, particularly when he wanted to ask me something about his work. But I had seven other students to work with in that class, and Victor's constant interruptions made it impossible for me to give the other students the help they needed. Since Victor could write, and he could understand why I couldn't always respond to him immediately, we agreed to use the following procedure: when I was working with another child or children, Victor would write his questions in a small notebook to be kept on top of his desk specifically for this purpose. When I finished working with a particular child or group, I would check in with Victor and go over any questions in his notebook before going on to work with other children.

Victor followed this procedure well, and the situation improved immediately. However, there were times when this strategy was inadequate, and Victor still became upset at not having immediate access to me. Therefore, we worked on a back-up strategy. When use of the question notebook was not enough, Victor was to change to a particularly soothing activity selected just for such times. Victor hit on the name "Upset Comforter" for this. His first Upset Comforter was coloring in a United Nations flag book that indicated exactly what colors should be used on all parts of each flag. This exactitude fit well with his need for certainty. With some prompting, Victor soon learned to recognize when it was time to get out his Upset Comforter. This was a strategy that he brought with him to his mainstream school and explained to his new classroom teacher the following year.

Pivotal Response Treatment is only one of the naturalistic behavioral strategies that has come to the fore in recent years, backed by supportive data on effectiveness. Incidental teaching is another naturalistic ABA approach. In this approach, the child's individual objectives and instruction are embedded in age-appropriate and developmentally appropriate activities. A preschool program for children on the spectrum that uses incidental teaching as a major strategy might look to an outsider much like a mainstream preschool program. What this more naturalistic behavioral strategy shares with more traditional ABA programs is ongoing assessment and record keeping, clearly delineated learning objectives based on that assessment, and the implementation of carefully planned instructional experiences and strategies closely tied to those objectives. Incidental teaching may look easy to do, but unless this approach is implemented with a high degree of care and skill, it will not be much more effective than a typical preschool would be in working with children on the autism spectrum.

Verbal Behavior (Sundberg and Partington 1998), which has become popular in recent years, is a naturalistic behavioral approach that focuses on establishing communication. It begins by looking at what the child wants in the natural environment and then teaching him or her how to request it. The child and the therapist sit on the floor, and the materials used are items the child enjoys. Parent training in the use of Verbal Behavior in the home is a major component of this approach. One of the professionals who has helped popularize this approach through many workshops is Vincent Carbone, who operates the Carbone Clinic in Valley Cottage, New York.

Many programs that refer to their approach as "eclectic" rely heavily on group instruction. This reliance may seriously reduce their effectiveness with children who have not yet broken the language code and still perceive the communications of others largely as a stream of meaningless sounds. A consistent, cohesive, and intensive individualized approach for helping these children acquire receptive language and an expressive language system is critical.

Some time ago I observed a class for five- to seven-year-old children with autism in a public school. Virtually all instruction was delivered in a group. The teacher was a dedicated person who spent a good deal of time planning and preparing materials. She would have been an excellent teacher for children with mild disabilities, but I doubt that her instructional efforts had much positive effect on most of the students in that class. The one child who had some receptive and expressive language, who could imitate and follow directions, seemed to be benefiting to some extent. He knew when the teachers were singing about him. He could retrieve the word card with his name on it when asked to do so. He could move his hands round and round like the wheels on a bus when a song about that subject was being sung, and he could hold up his fingers to match the words of another action song. The other children did not respond at all, apparently absorbed in their own worlds. From time to time an assistant teacher would guide a child's passive hands in motions matching the words of a song or would point to an item of the child's clothing, but there was no indication that the child understood what any-thing meant.

I watched this happen also in several preschool special education pro-grams where group instruction was the primary format. In spite of the hard work of conscientious teachers, precious learning time was being wasted. I asked one of these teachers what approach she was using. She informed me that she used "an eclectic approach."

Treatment and Education of Autistic and Related Communication-Handicapped Children, or TEACCH, is the North Carolina statewide comprehensive intervention system that has been providing a variety of services to individuals with autism and their families across all age groups since the 1970s. TEACCH operates an extensive training program for professionals, and the TEACCH model is being implemented in many areas of the country as well as other parts of the world. The primary edu-cational goal of TEACCH is to increase students' level of skill so that they will fit as comfortably as possible into the adult world, while respecting the "culture" of autism. "Recovery" is not a term used in this system. While ABA programs are generally based on the premise that the child must overcome autistic characteristics, in the TEACCH model the child is provided with an educational environment designed to accommodate the characteristics of children with autism.

A TEACCH classroom makes use of many visual organizers, including color-coded cues, because visual processing is a strength of so many chil-dren with autism. Areas for special activities have clear boundaries. There are picture or picture-word schedules for individual children and for the class. Individual work systems are organized to capitalize on the child's affinity for routines and to maximize independent functioning. Spon-taneous functional communication is the language goal of TEACCH, and alternative modes of communication such as pictures, manual signs, and written words are used when speech is particularly difficult for the child. Such strategies neutralize or counterbalance deficits common in children with autism and thus minimize behavioral problems. While the TEACCH model uses individual instruction for some new skills, group instruction is a major format.

So, parents may ask, what's the bottom line? How effective is a TEACCH approach? This is not an easy question to answer. Unlike the Young Autism Project model, which served a small and select group of children with autism, TEACCH is open to all children with autism spectrum disorders in the state of North Carolina. In addition, the TEACCH model is implemented in different settings such as mainstream classrooms and special classes. Over the years TEACCH has used a variety of measures to evaluate its effectiveness, including parent reports and rate of institutionalization. This latter measure was appropriate in the 1970s, when the TEACCH model began; today it is no longer a relevant outcome variable. Another outcome measure is parent satisfaction. A survey conducted by TEACCH in the late 1970s found that most parents were very satisfied with the services provided to their children and families, as they appear to be on some recent evaluations of TEACCH services. But the outcome measures that parents want to know about today are indices of children's performance.

The available performance data for children served by TEACCH after the 1970s come largely from studies focused on stability of IQ (Lord and Schopler 1989a, 1989b) rather than on the effects of treatment per se. Based on these studies, Catherine Lord and Eric Schopler report that substantial increases in IQ are common among children first evaluated at ages three or four, with the largest change found among children who were nonverbal and had IQ scores in the 30–50 range. These three-year-olds gained a mean of 22–24 points by age seven, while the four-year-olds gained an average of 15–19 points by age nine. However, most of these children still had IQs in the range considered to indicate mental retardation. Moreover, while a substantial number of children had increases of 20 points or more in IQ, decreases of this magnitude were found with equal or greater frequency among children first assessed after age three. Some more recent data tend to support the idea that TEACCH is more effective than programs with no specific approach guiding them (Mesibov, Shea, and Schopler 2004); but the data reported are too limited to allow conclusions to be drawn with any degree of certainty.

Although TEACCH doesn't have outcome data pointing to near-normal functioning, I thought again of Chris, the fourteen-year-old on the Lovaas videotape who had made only modest progress. Had Chris been in the TEACCH system, his mother wouldn't have spent two years teaching him to set a table. The TEACCH program helps students acquire functional work skills, and the TEACCH system has well-developed, supported work programs for people like Chris. It also has all kinds of family support services for people like Chris's mother, and Chris might have expanded his life experiences and skills in a TEACCH summer camp with other adolescents. A mother who was attending the Autism Society of America conference in 1995 explained to me that she returned to North Carolina when her son reached adulthood because the state in which she had been living for several years did not provide the variety and quality of services to adults with autism that the TEACCH system did. Her son now had a job he loved because of TEACCH, which found the job, trained him for it, and provided enough ongoing supervision to ensure that he would not lose it.

One major difference in overall strategy separating Lovaas-type programs and TEACCH is the different values these approaches assign to either accommodating the child's autistic characteristics or waging an all-out war against them. This is not a one-time decision. Decision points on this issue continue to present themselves throughout the child's educational treatment. I faced such decision points with Victor when he was my student. Victor was almost ten and had been receiving treatment for about five years when one such point arose.

The science unit the class had been pursuing for almost two weeks was the prediction, measurement, and reporting of weather. As the most academically able student in this class, Victor kept our daily weather records. Each morning when he entered the classroom he took my copy of the New York Times, *turned to its weather page, and recorded on the chalkboard both the previous day's weather report and the predicted weather for the current day. The class then used this information in a variety of ways. One morning on my way to work, I noted that my bus was about to leave as I reached the corner where I usually boarded after buying a newspaper. My choice was to buy the paper and miss the bus or forego the newspaper and catch the bus. I caught the bus.*

When Victor entered the classroom that morning expecting to find the New York Times *on my desk but didn't, he was extremely upset. I had been ready to suggest that he borrow the* Times *from the teacher next door (whom I had prepared for this request), but the suggestion came too late. For the next three hours until lunchtime Victor cried and screamed. I had not adequately accommodated his autistic difficulty in coping with unexpected events and changes in routines. But it was clear that the normal world would not abide by Victor's need for sameness. If he was to live in this world, he would have to learn to adapt to its unpredictability. Teaching Victor (and other students) to do so became the next instructional unit for the class and Victor's individual curriculum unit for many weeks to come.*

We focused on the idea that there are multiple ways to accomplish the same goal, and we practiced doing this in different situations, starting with the weather unit. I set the following question before the class: Suppose I were to forget to bring the Times *one day next week. How else could you get information about the weather? No one responded. I can think of one way, I said. Who else in the school has the* New York Times? *With this prompt Victor caught on, and in the next few days we borrowed the* Times *and other newspapers from various staff members. My next question to the class: Suppose one day no one had a newspaper. How else could we get a weather report? This time the prompt was not as useful, but we spent the next few days listening for the weather report on the radio, using the telephone to get the weather report, and going outside with a thermometer to record the temperature ourselves. Victor's homework was to listen to the weather report during the evening news. To make sure that Victor could make use of what we had been doing, I set one more question before him: Suppose I come in tomorrow without the* Times. *What would you do for your morning weather record? Victor went down the list of all the possible alternatives he could try. The next morning I "forgot" to bring the newspaper, and Victor coped beautifully.*

From that point on, each time Victor appeared to be falling into an unvarying routine, we went back to our study of alternative menus for reaching a particular goal. Had I continued to accommodate Victor's need for inflexible routines, he probably would have continued to have great difficulty coping in mainstream settings. Had I just insisted that he adjust, Victor's behavior might have deteriorated significantly. This balance between accommodation to autistic needs and adaptation to the expectations and demands of mainstream society must be handled with great care.

More than thirty years ago a mother faced this same decision about accommodating or battling against autistic characteristics and wound up using both strategies in her successful struggle to help her son become more like his typically developing peers. Accommodation took the form of removing all breakable or throwable objects and furniture from the home to reduce his violent behavior, but she fought against her son's insistence on sameness by systematically changing the arrangement of the remaining furniture and household routines, not allowing her son's protests and tantrums to deter her. To deal with her son's refusal to wear clothes, this mother purchased the few clothing items that appeared to attract him, and he began wearing one item continuously until he entered kindergarten and accepted the idea that he had to dress for school (Gajzago and Prior 1974).

COMBINING APPROACHES

Many families with ample financial resources use combinations of approaches with their children. Catherine Maurice implemented a Lovaas program with both her children, but they also received developmentally based speech/language therapy three times a week. Other children who attend preschool programs using a behavioral approach receive occupational therapy after school hours and may also be on special diets. One study of children in ABA programs found that parents used an average of seven additional types of treatments for their children (Smith and Antolovich 2000).

Some strong advocates of ABA attempted to stop this practice by denigrating all interventions other than ABA or by asking parents to make commitments not to use any treatments in addition to ABA. Some years ago I sat at a conference table with four sets of parents whose children were receiving ABA services from a highly regarded center that required such a commitment. All of those parents, who had ample financial resources, admitted to hiring speech/language therapists privately to work with their children after school hours using nonbehavioral approaches; three sets of those parents admitted to privately hiring occupational therapists as well. These parents recognized that ABA might not be the full answer.

The practice of combining intervention treatments has become widespread in the past few years for those families who can manage the work and expense required to make such arrangements. Some of these determined and dedicated parents, such as Lynn Hamilton and Christina Adams, reported clearly noticeable improvement in their children when selected treatments were added to the ABA menu. Moreover, sometimes even parents who are devoted to ABA conclude that it's time to try a different approach, particularly if the ABA treatment that had been used focused heavily on discrete trial instruction. This is what Lynn Hamilton concluded at one point:

> About two and a half years into ABA treatment, Ryan became increasingly aggressive and agitated during therapy sessions. He ran away when the therapist came into our home and was becoming more downcast daily. . . . our ABA consultant . . . realized Ryan was burned out with drills and desperately needed a change. Starting that day, Dr. Sallows stopped drills and initiated some of Greenspan's floor time methods with Ryan. For nine months we did no drills but focused on interacting with Ryan. . . . Ryan's behavior changed dramatically. Within weeks we regained our happy boy, and after the nine months we reinstated drills, this time with very positive responses. . . . I believe Greenspan's techniques were the right approach for our son at that time. However, I also believe that this method wouldn't have worked for Ryan in the beginning. He needed the structured learning in bite-size pieces that ABA offers. (Hamilton 2000, 239)

With some children, the point at which they need something other than ABA with a heavy dose of discrete trial teaching comes much sooner, as it did with Jonah:

> Jonah is now fighting for control at every turn. . . . he seemed to deliberately ignore or delay any requests I gave him lately. . . . And we've noticed that his anxiety's up too. . . . Hank reports that Jonah simply doesn't want to work the way he used to: the obliging, excited little boy of the first six months is gone. Now he tunes out, rolls on the floor, blows spit bubbles, talks silly, or simply refuses to look at the therapists. . . .

I remember in months past when I asked Hank, "Do you think he might be getting burned out?" Now I feel that they've created a child who won't even put on his socks without a battle, and I'm furious. . . . My cries to Hank are finally heard: pure table time is a thing of the past. Jonah can now learn from the environment, come up with his own ideas. . . .

After a few weeks of refusal, we sail into a clear patch of great therapy. He is so happy. (Adams 2005, 212–13, 247, 249–50)

Parents have been combining approaches in several different ways. One way is to use a developmental relationship-based model in the home to supplement the ABA approach used by professionals; another way is to select an approach that combines developmental strategies and behavioral procedures, such as Pivotal Response Treatment. Still another way is to insist that the approach being used be modified, as was done for Jonah, or be temporarily replaced, as was done for Ryan. What we need to keep in mind, however, are data showing that programs often referred to as "eclectic"—that is, programs that claim to incorporate a variety of strategies without having a clearly defined approach and staff skilled in implementing those strategies—often do not have a track record of good outcomes.

The Delaware Autistic Program combined strategies from several approaches, but the core of its model with young children who entered without speech was the Picture Exchange Communication System. PECS is a language training system developed, field tested, and implemented by Andrew Bondy and Lori Frost at the Delaware program. PECS has gained widespread acceptance as a bridge to speech for young children with autism.

Many children with autism have good visual skills but great difficulty in processing and producing speech. Thus, both manual communication and picture or picture-word systems of communication have been introduced when young children make very little progress in acquiring and using speech functionally. Manual communication, or sign language, has limited utility outside the classroom and home except in the deaf community, and in actuality most young children with autism acquire only a handful of signs (although even a few signs may have considerable value as a beginning). PECS may have greater utility for young children who do not acquire functional verbal communication for some time. Lack of an effective communication system is associated with increased tantrums, aggression, and even self-injury.

The Delaware Autistic Program didn't wait until children failed to respond to instruction. Its first language goal with the 80 percent of children who entered preschool programs without functional speech was to encourage each child to initiate communication and to do so within the contexts of social activities and play. (This starting point differs markedly from Lovaas-type behavioral programs, which focus initially on the production of speech sounds and word approximations along with the recognition of object names.) The child was taught to request desired items and activities by handing the adult a card with the picture of the item or activity on it. When the child did so, he or she was immediately rewarded by receiving that item or being allowed to engage in that activity.

Some parents worried that the introduction of any communication system other than speech would interfere with the acquisition of speech. Not so, says Andrew Bondy, former administrator of the Delaware Autism Program. Of the twenty preschoolers started on PECS from 1987 to 1992 who stayed in the Delaware Autism Program for more than two years, fourteen (70 percent) began using speech alone for communication, while another three (15 percent) used a combination of speech and PECS; only three children failed to acquire functional speech (Bondy and Frost 1994). Furthermore, many children are able to begin using PECS on the first day it is introduced, thus eliminating another long period when they continue to lack any effective means of communication. Today PECS is used widely in programs with a variety of basic approaches.

INCLUSION

The most dramatic movement in special education in the late 1980s and 1990s was the drive to include students with severe disabilities in the mainstream of education. This change was bolstered by the provision in federal education law that students with disabilities should be educated in the least restrictive environment appropriate to their educational needs. That clause was used in the early 1980s to support the shift of students from special schools to regular neighborhood schools and to limit the number of special education students with mild to moderate disabilities who were placed in special classes. By the late 1980s, the inclusion movement had attracted significant numbers of parents of children with severe disabilities; and school systems, prodded by the federal government, began to provide opportunities for such children to be included in the educational mainstream.

Why would the parents of a student with a severe disability want that child to be in a class with typical children? For several reasons, including the fact that normally developing children can be excellent role models and teachers. A child who can learn by observing other children will learn many desirable ways of acting and doing things from typical peers. Is this really relevant to educating children with autism? readers may wonder. It certainly is for at least some children.

Inclusion matches the dreams of parents of children with autism. They want their children in pre-kindergarten or kindergarten, feeding the dolls, building bridges, painting pictures, sharing and trading trucks with other children, and participating in "show and tell"—not sitting in classrooms where the silence is punctuated mostly by loud voices of teachers and occasional scripted phrases from children; where the curriculum may revolve around "point to red," "put with same," "touch circle," "what's your name?"; and where children say little or nothing to one another unless specifically prompted to do so.

Parents see the richness of programs for typical children, and they want some of that for their own children. The critical questions in this context are: When can this richness benefit a child with autism, and when will it be largely overwhelming confusion? How can we transform the richness that a child with autism may experience as a confusing maze into a situation that expands the child's experiences, boundaries, and adaptive capacities? Physical proximity to typically developing children does not ensure that this will occur, and mainstream teachers do not find it easy to support the special needs and goals of children with autism. It's easier when the child comes with some skills in communication and play, and when there is an adult who knows the child well to help with the tough times. When this is not the case, it may take an inordinate amount of determination, dedication, and skill to make this experience beneficial for the child with autism.

A mother of two children with autism faced a dilemma. She was undecided about the best educational course for one of her children. Both children were in a preschool program for children with autism that used a behavioral approach with one-to-one instruction. This mother felt very good about the progress of one child there, the one who had initially been less connected and responsive; but she wasn't sure about the benefits for her other child, who had always been more social and had shown few stereotyped behaviors before entering this program. Now that daughter was exhibiting more of such behaviors. Was she imitating the other children? the mother wondered. And if so, shouldn't she be in a program where children were doing things that would be helpful to her? Should she be moved to an early childhood special education program with children who did not have autism so that she could observe other children who communicated and played together? Would her daughter do better in a typical preschool class with a one-to-one aide and speech/language therapy? Given her daughter's continuing difficulty in understanding speech, how much would she get out of the group instruction dominant in these programs? Many parents face such decisions, and there is no one answer that is always "correct."

Sometimes the decision about inclusion is simplified because an available program has inclusion built into it. LEAP is such a program. Learning Experiences: An Alternative Program for Preschoolers and Parents was located in Pittsburgh, Pennsylvania, when it was established in 1981 as a federally funded model for the integration of typical children and children with autism. It is currently based in Denver, Colorado. While experimenting with different class sizes and groupings, this program settled on classrooms with ten or eleven typically developing children and three or four children who had autism spectrum disorders. The children, ages three to five, were at the preschool three hours a day, and parents were offered a skills training program and support group meetings.

Activities specifically designed to facilitate language, social interactions, and adaptive behavior in the students with autism supplemented the program's developmentally based early childhood curriculum. A variety of strategies were used to accomplish the program's objectives, including naturalistic teaching tactics such as incidental teaching, direct instruction with reinforcement, peer modeling, and use of dramatic play teaching scripts. One strategy designed particularly well by this program is peer-mediated learning. This involved training typical students to use facilitative strategies in interactions with their classmates on the spectrum across a variety of situations, including play episodes in which two or three typical students were paired with a classmate who had autism.

Research during the first twelve years of LEAP's operation showed that after two years in the program children had usually achieved a significant reduction in autistic characteristics and marked improvement on measures of intellectual development and language. Of the children with autism or PDD-NOS who spent two years in the program, twenty-four out of fifty-one were later enrolled in regular education classes; and some of these children had been enrolled in neighborhood kindergartens without any reference to their prior diagnosis (Strain, Kohler, and Goldstein 1996).

LEAP is an exceptionally well designed program that was directed by highly skilled professionals. It combines naturalistic approaches with creative strategies for systematic teaching. Its outcomes are not likely to be duplicated by other programs with less carefully developed and researched instructional programs. Nor are its achievements likely to be matched by programs with less favorable structural supports such as class size and ratios of typical children to children with autism. What LEAP demonstrated clearly is that a Lovaas-type behavioral model is not the only approach that can produce good outcomes in young children with autism, and that under certain conditions the integration of typical preschoolers and children with autism can be highly productive.

OTHER INTERVENTION STRATEGIES

Greenspan's DIR model is not the only relationship-based approach being used widely with children on the autism spectrum. Relationship Developmental Intervention (RDI) was designed to address the core problem of reciprocal social interactions that is one of the defining characteristics of autism spectrum disorders. Since Steven Gutstein introduced RDI in his book *Autism Aspergers: Solving the Relationship Puzzle* in 2000, interest in this approach has grown rapidly. It has continued to grow with the publication of two additional books and with training workshops offered all over the country, although thus far only one research study has been published on RDI.

This intervention approach does not address all the needs of children with autism. In fact, Steven Gutstein, its chief creator and disseminator, acknowledges that RDI might not be the only treatment needed for a child on the autism spectrum; and RDI makes no particular effort to address delays or difficulties in the acquisition of verbal language. The rapid growth of RDI is probably a testament to the poor track record of many traditional ABA programs and social skills training programs in helping children on the spectrum establish reciprocal interactions and strong relationships with more than a handful of family members and other adults. RDI offers parents hope that their child will experience joy, spontaneity, and true friendships.

Social Stories is an important strategy for addressing problems in social awareness in children and adolescents on the autism spectrum. The basic premise of this strategy is that when children and adolescents become more aware of the social expectations of varied situations—that is, what constitutes appropriate behavior and how their own behavior can be modified to meet those expectations—some of the persistent problems that appear to reflect noncompliance will be reduced (Gray 1995). A *social story* is usually a simple short story that highlights the expectations for behavior in a specific type of situation in which the child's or adolescent's behavior has been inappropriate. It also describes how the behavior affects others, and it often ends with a commitment from the individual to try to modify his or her behavior in a specific way.

Social stories are read with the child multiple times before or during relevant situations and activities. Research data support the effectiveness of Social Stories in decreasing behaviors that impede both learning and social acceptance. The Social Stories strategy has been incorporated into many programs for children on the autism spectrum and in particular by programs that serve students with Asperger syndrome.

Functional Behavioral Assessment (FBA) and behavior intervention plans are strategies for dealing with behavior that might be called challenging, interfering, or impeding—behavior such as tantrums or meltdowns, which are the bane of teachers and parents and which are often used as a rationale for keeping children out of the mainstream of schools. These strategies were developed and are implemented from within a framework of positive behavior support (Carr et al. 2002). FBA is based on the premise that behavior has a communicative function and that in order to change behavior that interferes with goals and objectives, the message encoded in the behavioral communication must be understood and respected.

Functional behavioral assessment is the first step in this process. It involves learning more about the conditions and factors that are associated with triggering and sustaining the impeding behavior and then formulating a behavioral intervention plan to reduce such behavior. What makes this approach "positive" is that it does not rely on "blaming the victim," that is, the child with autism, but rather "recognizes the relationship between behavior and environment" and therefore focuses on providing the supports, skill development, and modifications of settings and situations that would lessen the child's need for such behavior (Crimmins et al. 2004).

Since 1997 federal special education law, the Individuals with Disabilities Education Act (IDEA), has required school district teams that are responsible for developing Individual Education Programs (IEPs) to conduct functional behavioral assessments of problem behavior that interferes with learning and to implement behavior intervention plans with positive supports based on knowledge derived from the FBA.

In the 1987 *Handbook on Autism and Pervasive Developmental Disorders,* Patricia Mirenda and Anne Donnellan recommended a marriage of different curricular approaches, each contributing its particular area of strength. To a certain extent, this is what is happening today. Many different types of programs are incorporating individual schedules, visual organizers, social stories, and incidental teaching. More traditional ABA programs are incorporating PECS (or signing), Pivotal Response Treatment, incidental teaching strategies, and positive behavioral supports. Instead of focusing on how many pictures of objects a child can name, these programs are beginning to focus more on how many object names a child uses in communicating during everyday activities.

A funny thing seems to be happening out there in the world of educational therapeutic treatment of children with autism. Common elements are appearing in approaches that were once very different, even antagonistic, as programs learn and borrow from each other. Professionals seem more willing to acknowledge that maybe they haven't had all the right answers. In their 2005 book on Pivotal Response Treatment, the Koegels discuss strategies to elicit communication that are very similar to some presented by Stanley Greenspan and Serena Wieder in their 1998 book on the special needs child. The more gentle hand long espoused by programs based on a developmental approach has been creeping into ABA programs. The current naturalistic ABA approaches lend themselves better to meeting relationship-based goals than did the earlier traditional ABA approaches. Relationship-based interventions and skill-based interventions are no longer viewed by most professionals or parents as necessarily incompatible or mutually exclusive.

What ABA approaches did better than most other intervention programs was to document outcomes, both short-term and long-term. Very few other approaches or models collected outcome data. While there are many justifications for this lack—including the time and cost required to measure outcomes and follow up with children—this is information that parents feel they need in making decisions that may significantly affect their children's futures. One of the major reasons parents flocked to programs using Lovaas-based approaches in the 1990s was the outcome data he published. Parents who have options are no longer willing to take the word of a professional that his or her approach is very effective; nor are they satisfied with research that provides only narrowly based short-term data. They are saying, "Show me. My child's whole future is at stake, and it's too precious to entrust to some professional's say-so. What data do you have to support your claim of effectiveness?" Program directors and researchers should heed this message.

Educational treatment of children with autism has come a long way but is still only moderately effective for many children. To a significant extent, this reflects the fact that education is not a cure or even the optimal treatment for the neurobiological differences that underlie the conditions currently called autism. Other factors contributing to the modest effects of educational treatment for some children with autism are undoubtedly poor implementation of approaches and poor matches between the learning needs of particular children and the instructional strategies used in the programs that serve them.

According to a U.S. Government Accountability Office report of January 2005 on the special education of children with autism, almost 120,000 such children between the ages of six and twenty-one were receiving these services in 2002. That number is likely to increase substantially as the upsurge of children diagnosed with autism spectrum disorders between 1997 and 2005 is reflected in data from school systems. We have to provide better educational intervention services to these students. There are too many school administrators and teachers who do not understand the special needs of children with autism spectrum disorders, and too many inappropriate school placements are being made. Too many school programs are so "eclectic" that no instructional strategies are implemented with the intensity, consistency, and skill needed. Too many school systems are not receptive to moving children with autism into inclusive settings along with the specialized supports they are likely to need. School districts are paying too little attention to meeting the needs of children with Asperger syndrome. We don't know enough about how to match or tailor intervention approaches to best meet the needs and learning capacities of individual children on the autism spectrum. And we are undoubtedly "losing" children with autism who appear to have limited potential because we have not adequately helped them to acquire a communication system.

There is no room for complacency in the battle against autism. The tools we have to work with today are effective only when wielded with what Raun Kaufman, a young man who used to be called autistic, referred to as "passionate relentlessness."

7 Whatever Happened to Equal Opportunity?

Intensive one-to-one teaching for developmentally disabled children starting at the age of 2 should be an entitlement.

(Ivar Lovaas, quoted in Advocate *1994, 21)*

In the mid to late 1990s, in-home programs began springing up all over the country for preschoolers diagnosed with autism. Most of these programs were derived from the UCLA Young Autism Project model. After hearing about the "47 percent recovery rate" reported by Lovaas, parents began rejecting the preschool special education programs that school districts offered; or they accepted these programs initially but wanted to change to an in-home Lovaas-based model when their children showed little or no obvious improvement after a few months in special education. These parents were so determined not to allow anything to interfere with their children's progress toward recovery that they marshaled all their resources to pay for in-home services themselves at the outset and then fought for reimbursement later.

Of course, only some families could gather the money to pay for an intensive in-home program when reimbursement was questionable and at best far down the road. Not families whose income was only slightly above the poverty level; not families of five living on the salary of a firefighter or a teacher, no matter how much they wanted such treatment for their child. Even for the upper-middle-income families of many lawyers and doctors, the costs could be staggering, but those were the families who could and did stretch enough to undertake the expense of forty-hour-a-week in-home programs.

What were the costs? The UCLA Clinic for the Behavioral Treatment of Children offered training workshops to families to enable them to set up their own in-home programs based on the Young Autism Project model. The clinic recommended an initial two-to-three-day workshop, with a follow-up workshop every three or four months. The fees charged by the UCLA clinic in 1996 were $1,700 plus airfare, ground transportation, hotel, and $30 per diem for the two-day workshop; $2,300 plus the other charges for three days. Added to these workshop charges were the costs of ongoing direct instruction and additional fees for telephone and videotape consultations. A panelist at the April 1995 Westchester conference on behavioral approaches to autism (described in chapter 5) estimated the total cost of implementing the Lovaas in-home program as $3,500 to $4,000 a month, that is, $42,000 to $48,000 per year. Other families in New York City identified yearly expenditures for their preschool children at $40,000 to $60,000 during the mid to late 1990s.

But what about families whose annual income was less than $50,000, a category that includes a large segment of the American population, and parents who don't have extended family who can give or lend them money? What about their children's progress toward "recovery" or "best outcome"? What about single-parent families where that parent must work and try to juggle the coordination and monitoring of an in-home program as well as its cost? The UCLA Young Autism Project model and similar programs worked best when the family was generously endowed with several kinds of resources: money, intelligence, emotional resilience, and a good natural support system made up of friends, neighbors, and relatives.

School districts had little experience with supporting in-home programs in the 1990s and were much more comfortable with school-based programs. Yet in-home programs for young children have a long history. They began expanding in the late 1960s and early 1970s, with a focus on the prevention of school problems in children then labeled "disadvantaged," many of whom had IQ scores in the borderline or mildly retarded range. Thus, the Young Autism Project model was hardly the earliest in-home model for preschool children who were recognized as needing extra in-home supports. School districts rarely took part in these in-home programs, which drew support from a combination of sources other than state and local public education funds. Federal education laws passed between 1975 and 1990 began to change this picture dramatically, in the process easing the financial burden on families.

School systems that cannot provide appropriate education for children with disabilities ages three to twenty-one must pay for such educational services to be provided elsewhere. This was not always the case. Until the passage of the Education for All Handicapped Children Act of 1975, children with severe disabilities such as autism were often excluded from public education. With very few nonpublic options open to them, many of these children wound up without any educational services. The 1975 law dramatically changed that situation by introducing the concept of public responsibility for the education of *all* children, no matter how severe their disabilities. All children of school age were to receive a free and appropriate public education. Following the passage of this law, with prodding from judicial decisions in class action lawsuits, large school districts moved to include children with autism in their special education programs, while small school districts began to provide such services through intermediate or county programs. A great inequity had been redressed, and a severe service gap had been filled.

Until December 1986 federal law did not require states to provide services to preschool children with disabilities unless they also provided such services to preschool children who did not have disabilities, although states were given financial incentives to do so. Therefore, parents of children younger than five or six had no legal foundation from which to seek funding for in-home programs. The situation changed with the passage of the 1986 Amendments to the Education of the Handicapped Act, which held states responsible for supplying a free and appropriate education to children ages three to five who had handicaps.

Furthermore, a new section of this law introduced the idea of services to infants and toddlers from birth to age three and encouraged states to offer early intervention services. The Individuals with Disabilities Education Act (IDEA), the new name given to the Education of the Handicapped Act in 1990, included penalties for states that did not provide early intervention services to children under age three. By September 1994 all states had established systems of Early Intervention (EI) services. The legal foundation needed to allow parents to fight for the programs they wanted for their infants, toddlers, and preschoolers had been put into place.

By the late 1990s a new inequity had become apparent. It was not about the right to services; that battle had been won, at least for parents who knew how to find out what services their child was entitled to and how to go about getting them. The children of middle- and upper-income, well-educated parents were being identified and were receiving intervention services earlier and earlier. But many parents of toddlers and preschoolers—parents who were young and inexperienced and who had limited education and poor natural support systems—often did not recognize that something was going wrong in their child's development, that their child should be evaluated without delay, and that they were entitled to such an evaluation without any cost to the family. Federal special education law requires each state to ensure that all children with disabilities who are in need of special education services are identified and evaluated. Although the law mandates a comprehensive child-find system, a substantial number of children from very poor families are still not evaluated for an autism spectrum disorder until age four, five, or even six. This situation deprives children of an early start in the battle against the debilitating aspects of autism and thus weakens their odds of achieving good outcomes. It is a situation that needs significant attention and improvement.

The major battle about intervention in progress during the past ten years or so has been about the right to appropriate services, that is, about what is appropriate and who decides this. Put simply, when parents believe that the programs offered by school districts do not meet their children's educational needs, the parents with ample financial resources have been the ones most likely to be able to obtain alternative programs at public expense. Let's look at an example of how this might happen by returning to Westchester, where the conference featuring Ivar Lovaas was held in April 1995.

That conference was part of a fund-raising effort by a parent organization whose goal was to develop a school for children with autism that would use a behavioral framework. It had taken the parents about two years to reach that point. In 1993 several couples with young autistic children had come together to pool their resources with the objective of obtaining public funding for in-home programs using an applied behavior analysis approach. Some of these parents were already implementing and paying for such programs, sometimes after sampling and then rejecting special education preschool programs recommended by their local school districts. These parents had sought reimbursement from their health insurance companies but had not been successful. Now their target was the county of Westchester, whose approval was essential if in-home programs were to become an approved educational option for their children.

The parents knew what they were doing; some had legal backgrounds. They organized committees, lobbied politicians, and met with the relevant educational decision makers at state and local levels. They threatened lawsuits. The county began to show some interest and called a meeting for parents and directors of state-approved preschool programs. One agency agreed to sponsor the in-home programs. Its plan was approved by the county, and public funding was arranged. The agency added to its staff the "therapists" parents were already using, paying them as paraprofessionals for a total of thirty-eight hours a week per child. A trained behavioral specialist with certification in special education provided two hours of supervision each week. Having achieved the goal of publicly supported in-home Lovaas-type programs for their preschoolers, the parent organization moved on to other objectives, primarily the establishment of a school for children who continued to need intensive services after age five.

The Westchester story was a good story. It showed public education recognizing and supporting an option that might meet the needs of some children with autism better than any of the existing alternatives. A critical question that cannot be ignored is whether other citizens, less affluent and less knowledgeable about how to influence public systems, could have obtained equal consideration and a similar expansion of educational options for their children.

Let's look at a second group of parents who wanted exactly what the Westchester parents had won for their children. This second group of families did not live in an affluent suburban area. Most lived in Staten Island, with a few families coming from other boroughs of New York City. In January 1995 the first meeting of the Autism Advocacy and Outreach Group (AAOG), a recently revived parent organization, attracted close to a hundred parents and others. The first part of the meeting was spent airing complaints and voicing frustrations: parents had to scrape together every penny they had to pay for a few hours a week of in-home behavioral services, and they knew that this was insufficient; not enough schools in New York City were using this approach; and the public school system was not receptive to their pleas for such services. A determination to fight for what they considered their children's only hope was obvious. Then came a presentation by one of the mothers from the Westchester parent organization on the strategies that group had used to achieve its goals.

An attorney from New York Lawyers for the Public Interest was the speaker at the second AAOG meeting. This nonprofit law office had been designated as the protection and advocacy agency for people with developmental disabilities in New York City. (Under federal developmental disabilities laws dating back to the 1970s each state had to have a system to protect and advocate for the rights of persons with developmental disabilities.) This agency had agreed to work with the parents in AAOG to help them obtain appropriate services for their children. As a starting point, a letter had been sent to relevant persons within the public school system outlining the issues and objectives.

Over the next few months meetings were held with school district representatives. A proposal for specific new services was invited and submitted, but no new programs were initiated by the board of education either for preschool children or young school-age children at that time. Some nonpublic agencies providing special education services in New York City were, however, beginning to listen to parents; and in September 1995 a couple of behavioral programs for preschool children were started. But these were center-based programs; the quest for publicly funded, intensive, Lovaas-type in-home programs for preschoolers had not been successful. In the meantime, movement through legal pathways was slow, and parents became increasingly discouraged about being able to obtain the intensity of services that the Westchester families had secured.

In Westchester, as 1996 approached, the parent organization moved closer to opening its new behavioral school for children ages five and older. In New York City, parents who believed that public school classes for autistic students five and older offered no hope for their own children continued to hire private advocates to help them get approval for non-public school placements—that is, if they could afford the fees that such private advocates charged. And even then, the "victory" was sometimes of limited value because the number of nonpublic schools serving autistic children with the kind of program that the parents sought was very small.

A year after the Westchester conference on behavioral intervention in autism, a 1996 version of that conference—same sponsoring organization, same subject, same place, and some of the same speakers—was scheduled to take place. I was looking at the conference brochure, trying to decide whether to go. Instead, I picked up the telephone and called the African American mother from Brooklyn whom I had met at the conference the previous year. Her son was six by then, I realized. This time I reached her.

None of the promises of help she had received at the conference last year had materialized except for a parent outreach program. Her son was still in the same class in the same public school, doing about the same. Now she felt a new need to push for something else. Individual speech/language services would no longer be available to her son in the public school program he attended, this mother told me; all such services would be delivered to groups of students in the classroom. She was trying to find a private advocate or attorney whom she could afford to fight for her son's placement at a private school that used a Lovaas-type behavioral model. The advocate she had called would not talk to her without a $600 payment up front, which this mother didn't have. What this mother wanted for her son was some kind of a life, some kind of a future in which he could be productive and would have satisfying experiences. She didn't see him being helped toward that now.

What was happening in other parts of the country between the mid 1990s and the early years of the twenty-first century concerning the provision of in-home behavioral options for preschool children? An analysis of sixty-eight cases published between 1997 and 2002 that involved Individualized Education Programs (IEPs) for students with autism showed that most of those cases involved parental requests for intensive ABA in-home programs or for reimbursement of the costs of such programs (Etscheidt 2003). Parents won 43 percent of the cases, while the school district prevailed in 57 percent.

The activities just described focused on the educational treatment of children ages three and older. Since the end of the 1990s, however, there has been an explosion in the number of toddlers identified as having autistic disorder or PDD-NOS. The Individuals with Disabilities Education Act treats children from birth through age two differently than children three and older. It gives each state the right to choose the lead state agency for the provision of comprehensive, interagency services to infants and toddlers. Fewer than a third of the states chose the state education department; health agencies were most commonly selected.

While IDEA guaranteed that services to children ages three and older would be free to the parent, there was no such guarantee for children younger than three. States were given the right to establish sliding-scale fee structures for family payment if this practice was consistent with state law, although no state could deny services because of a family's inability to pay or charge any family for an initial evaluation or for program coordination. States have responded to this regulation in different ways.

Most states do not charge fees to families; others have cost-participation or sharing systems that require modest annual fees for families with incomes above a certain level. Payment for early intervention services must be sought from such sources as private health insurance and Medicaid before funds provided through IDEA may be used, unless this causes a delay in providing timely services to the child. States have also pursued different tactics in regard to that requirement. Some passed legislation to ensure that private insurance would cover early intervention costs up to a certain point (for example, $5,000 annually in Connecticut, Rhode Island, and Virginia); other states have made agreements to ensure that payments from private insurers would not count toward lifetime caps.

In-home services are the most common form of service delivery for infants and toddlers under IDEA, but the intensity of services provided to these young children has generally been low. In some states the norm was two hours a week, and children with autism or PDD-NOS who needed more hours of dedicated instruction often could get them only if their parents could pay for or provide the additional services themselves. The success of Westchester parents in gaining intensive services for preschoolers had not carried over to toddlers. In New York State, services to preschoolers fall under the jurisdiction of the New York State Education Department, while services to infants and toddlers are under the direction of the New York State Department of Health. Thus, parents had a different bureaucracy to deal with and a new battle to wage.

In early 1995 I spoke to an early intervention service coordinator in New York. Most infants and toddlers were receiving two hours a week of services, she told me, but some parents of two-year-olds with diagnoses of autism or PDD-NOS had pressed hard for more and were now getting up to eight hours of service. A year later I spoke to this coordinator again. Five or six lawsuits initiated by parents were now pending in New York City, she reported. The issue was intensity of services, that is, number of hours provided. The service limits had already been pushed upward, to a maximum of sixteen hours a week of in-home services, and a precedent had been established for children to receive combinations of center-based and in-home services that together exceeded twenty hours. The parents who had filed lawsuits wanted reimbursement for thirty-five to forty hours a week of in-home programs. To some extent the activities of parents with greater financial resources who paid for the in-home programs of their toddlers and then fought for reimbursement benefited parents with more limited financial resources as well. The legal actions of the wealthier parents led to an expansion of service hours for other families and stimulated the initiation of new programs for toddlers.

In the late 1990s the New York State Department of Health initiated a project to establish guidelines for early intervention services. The guidelines on autism, which were produced by a panel of experts, favored at least twenty hours a week of intensive, individual ABA services. Although these guidelines were not prescriptive, they supported parent requests for increased amounts of service and helped make New York one of the states with the most generous early intervention service provisions.

The picture just described of intervention services in the 1990s and at the beginning of the new century is now changing. The Westchester parents opened the school they had fought for and it exists today, as do a substantial number of other nonpublic schools for children with autism that receive public funding. Some of the children of the Staten Island parents now attend a school district program that uses a behavioral approach designed with parental input, and many school districts are either providing or funding ABA preschool programs.

The primary issue today is the intensity and quality of these services. One-to-one services for twenty-five or more hours a week are rarely offered to young children; the training of teachers and the aides or assistant teachers who work with them is often quite skimpy and inadequate; and supervision in public programs may well be provided by a special education teacher who has little training in working with children on the autism spectrum or with the particular approach being used. While parent advocacy centers for lower-income families exist, those parents who can afford to consult with highly experienced attorneys are still at a great advantage in obtaining IEPs with more intensive services or with the kind of supports that improve the chances of successful inclusion. Those parents also more often succeed in getting approval for private schools when they are not satisfied with the programs offered by the school district.

In a 2005 report the U.S. Government Accountability Office indicated that the estimated school district per pupil expenditure on a child with autism was $18,790 during 1999–2000. This was substantially more than the $6,556 per pupil expenditure for the typical student, but was it enough to offer the intensive and extensive services that were considered best practice for young children with autism and that might make a significant difference in the futures of these children? Shortly after the period referred to in that report a private school for children with autism opened in New York City, with cost to parents of $60,000 a year; that cost had risen substantially by the 2005–2006 school year. In 2005 a small charter school opened in New York City that was free for parents but received $60,000 a year in public funds for each of its students. These schools were able to offer state-of-the-art ABA programs that were consistent with the recommendations of the National Research Council.

The high costs of providing intensive educational intervention to young children with autism, together with the requirement in the "No Child Left Behind" federal law mandating that all teachers be highly qualified, have contributed to a movement within Early Intervention toward defining the family as the major deliverer of services. This shift is consistent with the current focus on family-centered teaching and teaching in natural environments. For children younger than three the home is the primary natural environment, and it makes sense to help parents acquire skills in facilitating their own child's development through interactions and activities in the home and the community. Furthermore, the Pivotal Response Treatment model used by the Koegels and the models used by other state-of-the-art centers for autism rely heavily on the family's involvement in providing intervention with the intensity needed.

But I have concerns about this development. Parents may acquire a high level of skill in supporting their child's development but not have the time or stamina to deliver learning support with the necessary consistency and intensity. Other parents, themselves limited by cognitive or emotional problems, may not be able to acquire the skills needed or may be unable to deliver them skillfully. Parents with sufficient resources will hire additional service providers privately to supplement the professionally delivered services from the EI system; or they may quit their jobs to devote virtually all their time to their autistic child; or they may hire a nanny or housekeeper to help them with other children and family chores so that they can give most of their time and attention to their autistic child. Families that are already stretched to the ends of their resources and coping abilities will not fare well unless support packages are created with much flexibility and with recognition of the greater service needs of these families. Otherwise we will be increasing inequity rather than lessening it.

Let's look further at the equity picture today by considering one family. A few months ago a mother wrote to me. She had four children younger than eight, including a six-year-old with autism. She desperately wanted to do right by her son, but she was approaching her wit's end. Her son had made good progress in his early intervention and preschool programs and was now in an inclusion kindergarten, where he was reportedly doing well most of the time. However, he was having meltdowns of increasing length and frequency at home, and his stereotyped behavior had increased both at home and in school. After one of her son's lengthy meltdowns this mother had fantasized about getting her son out of the home, but that was not the resolution she wanted.

I was not the first professional beyond the school system to whom this mother had reached out. She had contacted at least two other professionals that I knew of, including a highly regarded ABA specialist. That individual had recommended a thorough functional behavioral assessment and had given the mother the name of a private consultant skilled in such assessment. The cost of that assessment by this consultant was over $100 an hour. This family, with several other children to support, could not find any way to pay that cost.

IDEA requires a functional behavioral assessment for children with disabilities whose behaviors impede their own learning or that of others. Functional behavioral assessment is a problem-solving procedure designed to identify why a student engages in such behavior and what is likely to be effective in eliminating or reducing it. In this case, however, the school did not perform a functional behavior analysis because it did not consider the child to be presenting seriously challenging behavior in the classroom.

After I responded to this mother, she asked the school district for a meeting to review her son's IEP. As a result of that meeting more time was provided for a special education teacher to work with her son in his classroom, and counseling services aimed at social skill development were added. Neither of the additions to the IEP was likely to do much good, I thought, especially since the mother saw no evidence that either the special education teacher or the school counselor knew how to work with a child on the autism spectrum. Moreover, there was no attempt to help the mother understand how to deal with her son's meltdowns at home, which threatened the safety of his younger siblings as well as his mother's stability.

How would this situation have been different if this family had had greater resources? I asked myself. Resources include time and the supports that money can buy. A functional behavioral assessment would have been conducted, and a behavioral intervention plan would have been developed. The private consultant might have been used in an ongoing way to monitor the effectiveness of the behavior intervention plan, to suggest modifications as needed, and to assist the parents in implementing the plan in the home. This family would also have been able to consult with a medical specialist experienced in working with children on the autism spectrum, someone the mother could rely on to use good judgment in considering the need for medication if the behavior intervention plan did not prove sufficiently effective.

You may be thinking that this was a family living at the poverty level, headed by parents with limited education. It was not. This family was headed by bright, devoted, and hard-working parents with college degrees. Think about the children of families who do not have these positive factors operating.

Let's look at this question of equity from another angle, that of "Autism Mommies" and "Autism Super Mommies," concepts presented by Christina Adams in her book *A Real Boy* (2005). These parents may to a considerable extent be responsible for the reports about good outcomes that appear to be on the increase, even though some Autism Super Mommies have children who make only moderate progress.

Adams classifies parents into four categories. She refers to the largest category of parents as "Special-Needs Parents"—parents who accept whatever the service system offers. She designates the next largest group of parents as "the Upgrade Crowd"—parents who try to enhance the services that the school system offers, particularly when their child has made very little progress. Then there is a small category of "Autism Mommies," who do everything that has any remotely reasonable chance of helping their child, including twenty-five to thirty hours a week of in-home programs, in addition to a part-time special education class; special diets; and testing by various medical specialists.

Finally, Adams describes a very small category of "Autism Super Mommies"—parents with "a river of money and time, and a formidable brain," all devoted to their child and, at some point, to families of other children with autism. These Autism Super Mommies have in-home programs of forty or more hours a week, consult numerous professionals who possibly know something that might help their child, spend hours with therapists of various sorts, combine different intervention strategies or switch them at different points in their child's development, and create enchanting play areas to entice neighborhood children to interact with their child (2005, 189–90). They use only professionals who are considered highly skilled, if not at the very top of their fields of expertise. When these parents can't obtain the best services and as much service as they want at public expense, they pay for it with their own funds.

These parents are to be greatly respected both for their devotion to their own children and for the contributions they make to the overall field of autism. They are the driving force behind the recent upsurge of research into autism, the public awareness of autism, and the increased resources devoted to intervention for children with autism spectrum disorders. They also greatly improve their own child's chances at more typical development. All devoted parents would like to be able to do this, but most can't; all children with autism deserve this, but many don't receive it.

What can and should we do about this? We cannot turn low-income families into upper-income families, nor can we enable mothers of children with autism who must work to support their families to give up their jobs. We cannot provide mothers who have multiple young children and limited means with nannies so that they can spend more time meeting the needs of their autistic child. We cannot ensure that parents with limited educations will know how to get the most out of the available service systems. We cannot ensure that all families will be able to cope with the additional stresses associated with having a child with autism, nor can we guarantee that every family will have access to physicians who are knowledgeable about identifying and treating the special needs of children with autism. We cannot ensure that every child with autism has educational intervention that is appropriate and is delivered with a high level of skill. We cannot do these things, but it should be our goal to get as close as possible to achieving this level of care for all children with autism and their families. We should be figuring out how to improve our support systems to enable these families to give to and get for their autistic children more of the "good stuff" that Autism Mommies deliver.

Undoubtedly, the service picture for young children with autism today is much brighter than it was in the past, but it is still not bright enough. The years before age seven or so are critical years for battling the debilitating aspects of autism. Services that are skimpy will not do, and a society that values equal opportunity cannot afford to tolerate inequities that may have significant lifelong consequences. The tenor of the times does not favor new entitlements, so Lovaas's entitlement recommendation for intensive one-to-one teaching for all two-year-olds with autism, quoted at the beginning of this chapter, has little chance of being heeded. But steps need to be taken—by states, counties, and local educational authorities; by parents, individually and in organized groups; by disability advocacy organizations, by educators and medical professionals—to ensure that economic factors do not deprive some children with autism and their families of the skilled collaborators and intensive supports they need in the struggle to achieve a good future.

8 Some Thoughts on Alternative Treatments and Other Intervention Controversies

> Within minutes of coming home from the clinic that Thursday,
> I was on the phone, beginning to pursue Ryan's recovery.
>
> *(Hamilton 2000, 28)*

Because most children with autism don't "recover" or achieve near-normal functioning, and because many children with autism struggle for years against formidable challenges to their understanding and happiness, parents and professionals continue to search for better answers. The search for a cure for autism is over fifty years old, but this search has taken on powerful allies and major resources only since the late 1990s. False starts and detours have marked the way, along with optimism and "miraculous cures" that turned out to be less than miraculous and less than a cure.

Perhaps the most damaging detour was the belief that autism was caused by parental behavior toward the child, particularly by a mother's cold rejection. Leo Kanner, the child psychiatrist who first brought attention to the condition referred to as autism, inadvertently led the way into this detour. While Kanner believed that autism grew out of an innate inability to form relationships, he also referred to the "emotional frigidity in the typical autistic family" and to the "dramatically evident detachment, obsessiveness, and coldness that is almost a universal feature of parents of autistic children" (Eisenberg and Kanner 1956, 561). The view of autism as reflecting an inborn defect in relating did not fit the zeitgeist of the 1950s and most of the 1960s, an era that was permeated by psychoanalytic perspectives on child dysfunction. If autistic children were cut off from and nonresponsive to the significant others in their lives, it was assumed that this resulted from something the child had been deprived of, something parents should have done but didn't, or perhaps something parents shouldn't have done but did. The era of blaming parents for their child's autism was in full bloom.

What Kanner and other professionals did not consider was the process of reciprocal interaction—initiation and reinforcing response—that takes place between parents and their normally developing babies, and the effect on parents of having a nonresponsive child who is also difficult to understand and manage. Professionals also did not consider that the parental behavior they were witnessing might have been the end result of a long period of uncertainty, doubt, and stress about the child's development. (Still another hypothesis posed recently in light of growing evidence of genetic involvement in autism is that some of the parents of autistic children seen by Kanner might themselves have been mildly autistic or might have had Asperger syndrome.)

Given this view of autism as a form of emotional disturbance growing out of a lack of warm and loving care during the early years, psychodynamic treatment approaches dominated the 1950s and 1960s. In her 1964 book *Dibs in Search of Self,* Virginia Axline presented her young patient as a case in point, that is, as a child who had been cured through play therapy; and Bruno Bettelheim, the most notorious blamer of parents, claimed cures of children with autism through psychodynamic milieu therapy after separating children from their families. Many of Bettelheim's claims have been vigorously disputed, and Axline's success in using play therapy with "Dibs" was rarely replicated with severely impaired autistic children. It was a parent-professional, Bernard Rimland, who in his 1964 book *Infantile Autism* presented the evidence against psychogenic interpretations of autism so compellingly that a death knell began to sound for these views. At the same time, the search for an organic cause of autism gained much-needed vigor.

Good research is a time-devouring process. Small chunks of a problem are tackled one by one as hypotheses are generated and explored. As layers of information accumulate, researchers construct or modify theories to fit all the known pieces. The search for the organic or neurobiological underpinnings of autism has recently taken on new momentum. Bolstered by technological advances, research has begun to yield very promising clues. But cures or even highly effective treatments for autism tied to its neurobiological origins still appear to be a long way off. In the meantime, parents of autistic children wait impatiently and look elsewhere, grasping at promising possibilities.

Today's promising possibilities, most with minimal supportive evidence from careful research, are the treatment alternatives to which parents with resources are flocking and in which they invest not only their money but also their dreams. Lynn Hamilton (2000) pursued that dream through nineteen different types of interventions for her son Ryan. From a researcher's point of view, such parents are investing in hypotheses or educated guesses. From the parents' point of view, they can't afford to wait; the results of thorough research may come too late for their own children. Some years ago, I asked a psychiatrist who is highly regarded and widely published in the area of autism what he thought of using prednisone to treat children diagnosed with late-onset autism who had EEG patterns like those seen in Landau-Kleffner syndrome. "It's premature," he replied. He was right, particularly since that drug can have perilous side effects when used for more than a brief period; but to the parents of a child who has lost the ability to speak, to understand speech, and to participate in the joys of childhood, the risk might be considered worth taking.

Today's controversial alternative treatments may become the discarded guesses of tomorrow, but one or more of them may turn out to be an effective form of treatment for a substantial number of children with autism. In the meantime, using these treatments involves a balancing act, weighing risks against potential benefits. Supposed breakthroughs in treating autism are still appearing. Unfortunately, none has proven to be a major breakthrough for most children with this disorder.

Bernard Rimland has devoted most of his adult life to identifying and tracking possible treatments for autism. In the process, working out of the Autism Research Institute in San Diego, which he founded in 1967, he brought to the attention of parents and professionals many of the alternative treatments used during the past twenty years as well as today. He also personally championed several treatments whose efficacy he believed in but most other professionals did not.

Megavitamin therapy is an alternative treatment that Rimland has studied for over twenty years. He fervently believed in the value of vitamin B6 for a substantial proportion of the autistic population and still advocates supplementation with a combination of B6 and magnesium, preferably through a megavitamin formulated for this purpose. What such treatment achieved in about 35 to 50 percent of children with autism, according to Rimland, was improvement in attention and learning, along with decreases in hyperactivity and irritability.

Some recent research indicates that vitamin B6 may have a beneficial effect because it modulates the function of neurotransmitter enzymes. Abnormalities in this area, particularly high blood levels of serotonin, have been identified in a substantial number of children with autism; but very high doses of vitamin B6 can be quite harmful. Moreover, the research cited in support of vitamin therapy is not widely viewed as very convincing.

Of all the supposed breakthroughs of the late 1990s, secretin was the best publicized. This is what we've been waiting for, announced Bernard Rimland with much fanfare at a 1998 conference of the Autism Society of America. The reports by Rimland and Victoria Beck, the mother who first convinced a doctor to administer secretin to her three-year-old son and later told the world of his remarkable improvement, sent hundreds of desperate parents scurrying to find a doctor who would administer this substance.

Secretin is a hormone that is normally secreted in response to excess acidity in the stomach. It is used in the diagnosis of gastrointestinal disorders. Secretin appeared to have a beneficial effect on the gastrointestinal systems of some children with autism who have significant problems with the functioning of that system. Behavioral improvements were also noted in a few of these children, but behavioral improvement is not surprising when chronic physical problems such as diarrhea and its accompanying discomfort are eliminated. One early study of three children treated with secretin appeared to show substantial improvements in social interaction and language; however, that outcome was not found in later studies (Esch and Carr 2004).

Soon hundreds or perhaps even thousands of individuals with autism were being given this substance off-label, often at very high cost. This development led the National Institutes of Health to authorize several studies of secretin, and a number of other studies were also conducted around the country. The results of this research place secretin in the same category as supposed breakthroughs from earlier years: it may provide help to a tiny percentage of children with autism, while having little or no beneficial effect on the functioning of most children with this disorder. More research is needed on the prevalence of gastrointestinal disorders in children with autism and on the very small subset of children who seem to demonstrate improvement after receiving secretin.

The "Defeat Autism Now!" (DAN!) conference held in early 1995 was convened by Bernard Rimland. About thirty medical researchers participated by invitation. The conference produced a report on state-of-the-art alternative medical approaches to the treatment of autism, representing a consensus of the participants. Suggested interventions included vitamin supplementation, intravenous immunoglobulin, antifungal medication, and gluten-and-casein-free (GFCF) diets. (Gluten is a substance found in wheat and some other grains, and casein is a milk protein.) Each intervention was tied to the identification of a biological problem, with immune system dysfunctions and their effects highlighted. The conference report was followed in the fall of 2005 by another publication of the "Defeat Autism Now" project, *Autism: Effective Biomedical Treatments*, by

Jon Pangborn and Sidney Baker. That book describes and discusses virtually all the alternative biomedical procedures current at that time.

In the foreword to the book *Unraveling the Mystery of Autism and Pervasive Developmental Disorder,* in which Karyn Seroussi highlights the benefits of a gluten-and-casein-free diet for her son Miles, Bernard Rimland writes: "The salient message of this book is that parents who want to help their autistic children must look beyond traditional medicine for answers" (Seroussi 2000, 14). A substantial number of parents have reported marked decreases in their children's autistic behavior after a GFCF diet was instituted, and increases in such behavior with the reintroduction of wheat and dairy products. Karyn Seroussi tells of her own experience in listening to parents like Chris Braffet Delnat, whose son improved on the diet:

> When I started my son on the diet we were at the bottom of a downhill behavioral slide with nowhere else to turn. Andrew had been expelled from school for aggressive, uncontrollable behavior and I was with him the majority of the day, one-on-one just to keep him from hurting himself too badly. . . . he could maintain some semblance of composure only in the security of his own room. . . .
>
> My son has been gluten-and-casein-free for about a year now, and it has been the best year ever. He is no longer aggressive, ever, and no longer has wide and wild mood swings. His nocturnal bowel movements and the consequent feces smearing is gone . . . (Seroussi 2000, 69, 68)

No one disputes the fact that some children with and without autism are sensitive to casein or gluten; and a very small number of children may have undiagnosed celiac disease, an intestinal disorder that involves damage from foods containing gluten and may also include lactose intolerance. What is in dispute is whether there is a higher incidence of such problems in children with autism spectrum disorders and whether the GFCF diet has a significant beneficial effect on some of these children. Most of the current evidence that supports the use of GFCF diets is anecdotal or in the form of case studies; but some medical researchers have been listening to parents, and the possibility that the GFCF diet may benefit some children with autism is being tested in at least one well-designed research study supported by the National Institute of Mental Health.

The flyer from a local chapter of a disability agency announced a February 1996 presentation by a researcher, William Shaw, PhD. In bold lettering the flyer read, "Could fungal or bacteriological infections be involved in your child's attention deficit disorder or autism?" The flyer went on to ask, "Could your ADD/autistic child benefit from dietary changes and antifungal medication?" These questions are still being asked today. Not enough research has been done to convince most medical specialists concerned with autism that elevated levels of fungi or bacteria are involved in autistic behavior or that the recommended treatments will make a substantial difference in the learning or behavior of a significant number of individuals with autism. Virtually all evidence comes from anecdotal reports. Yet a number of parents are using antifungal medications such as nystatin and Diflucan, and some are reporting startling improvements in their children's behavior when such medication is added to their treatment regimen:

> After a series of allergy tests, blood panels, and the lab tests, we start Jonah on Nystatin. . . . As the days progress, we float into his best month yet. Week after week, he does amazingly well. Tantrums are down, say the teachers. Language is fantastic. Eye contact is better. Compliance . . . is excellent. . . . I've allowed myself to dream of his getting better, to hesitantly nod when others have said it will happen, but only now do I let myself feel it. . . .
>
> We are told to stop the Nystatin. . . . He's been taking it for four weeks and thriving. Now the neurologist wants us to go without it for at least a month. . . . Within three days, he starts to regress. . . .
>
> We go back on the Nystatin. It kicks in within four days, and a week later it's clear: Jonah is coming back. (Adams 2005, 122, 126, 131)

There is some evidence of immune system abnormalities in at least some children with autism. A number of research reports appear to support the idea that such differences may contribute to susceptibility to autism and to autistic characteristics. The role of immune system abnormalities in autism is currently a subject of mainstream medical research, with some funding for such studies provided by the National Institutes of Environmental Health Sciences and the U.S. Environmental Protection Agency. Much more investigation is needed in this area, but in the meantime, many parents are paying substantial sums of money for immunological evaluations and follow-up treatment. One treatment commonly associated with such testing is intravenous immunoglobulin therapy (IVIG). Only limited research data support this treatment, but anecdotal reports, such as the one that follows, entice desperate families into trying IVIG infusion.

> Following the infusion Peter developed a fever of 104 the first night. . . . The ensuing nine days he was somnolent and cranky. . . . Suddenly on the tenth day Peter emerged as a "new boy." He previously had no language and now is using appropriate language (i.e., "Momma, I wanna, donwanna. No. shoe, Santa") and increasingly articulate babbling, on a daily basis. His eye contact has improved dramatically. Previously he paid no attention to his cousin and now he initiates contact and play. He is now initiating hugs with his mom, where before he would only hug in response to his mom's approach. He is now having perfect poops for the first time in a long history of irritable bowel symptoms. His receptive language has taken a leap. He can be left ungated in rooms and will come when called and will walk with his mom without being held, whereas before he was wild. (Pangborn and Baker 2005, 126)

In response to the belief that childhood exposure to thimerosal, a form of mercury used in some vaccines, had triggered autism and that removal of excess mercury could reduce their children's autistic behavior, some parents have sought chelation therapy. This therapy has been used for some time with children who have been found to have very high levels of lead. Chelating agents or medicines help rid the body of the excessive heavy metals, which can cause neurological impairment and lead to problems in learning and attention. However, chelation therapy cannot undo any neurological damage that has already occurred as a result of heavy metals. It must also be used with great care as it can have dangerous side effects. To date, reports supporting the benefits of chelation therapy for children with autism come almost entirely from parents. Bernard Rimland, ever the champion of alternative treatments, states on the Autism Research

Institute web site that thousands of autistic children have demonstrated remarkable improvement with chelation therapy.

Another alternative treatment that was championed by Bernard Rimland is auditory integration training (AIT). AIT was popularized by the publication of the book *The Sound of a Miracle* (1991), written by the mother of a girl with autism. "A miracle" is the way Annabel Stehli described her daughter's response to AIT. Georgiana Stehli was diagnosed as autistic just before age three and entered an intensive educational treatment program a few months later, where her mother noted that she was making good progress. Still, at age eleven, Georgie was considered to be of borderline intelligence and too vulnerable and dangerous to live at home. Life in a residential setting was what professionals envisioned as her future. It wasn't a future her mother wanted any part of, so when she learned of a treatment for children with hyperaudition that held out the possibility of "recovery," Annabel Stehli pursued it.

She noted signs of improvement almost immediately after the brief treatment period. For the first time, Georgie wasn't afraid of certain sounds—the wind, ocean waves, or even people's voices. "The rain didn't sound like a machine gun anymore," Georgie stated in a television interview. She wanted to go out and play, began to make new friends easily, and began to take pleasure in conversation. Although much remained to be done, Georgie now wanted to become normal, asked for instruction in achieving this goal, and soaked up the instruction her mother gave her. Her IQ, which had been measured at 75 a year earlier, was now 97. Annabel Stehli felt that Georgie had been rescued.

What exactly is the treatment process that purportedly led to this dramatic improvement? And what was its effect on others with autism? The premise of AIT is that some of the characteristics of autism are a result of a sensory dysfunction and may involve hypersensitivity at certain sound frequencies, making some common sounds very painful to the autistic individual. (According to Bernard Rimland, about 49 percent of children with autism have symptoms of sound sensitivity.) The goal of AIT is to normalize the child's auditory input. In AIT a child or adult listens to modulated music through headphones for two half-hour periods a day over ten days, with certain sound frequencies filtered out. Why this should result in improved functioning is not clear.

Annabel Stehli believed so strongly in AIT that she devoted herself to spreading the word about this treatment through the Georgiana Institute, which was established for this purpose. While other parents have reported improvements following AIT, no "miracles" have been reported, nor anything approaching a miracle. Geraldine Dawson and Renee Watling (2000) reviewed the research literature on interventions designed to address sensory and motor impairments. They found that while sensory impairments are common in autism, controlled studies of auditory integration provide little or no support for this intervention strategy.

Sensory integration therapy may be thought of as an intervention approach that parallels AIT but that focuses on other types of sensory input. It is one of the major treatment approaches or strategies used by occupational therapists—health professionals who treat children and adults with motor and sensory motor problems. Sensory integration therapy is widely used in programs for children with autism, many of whom are assessed as having sensory motor difficulties. Nonetheless, researchers are skeptical about the value of sensory integration therapy, citing multiple weaknesses in the design of studies that claim positive results and multiple studies that found no benefit from this treatment. Why, then, is this form of treatment used so widely? One reason is that it seems intuitively right.

No one who reads Temple Grandin's first book, *Emergence: Labeled Autistic* (1986), or hears her speak of her childhood and adolescence will ever forget the machine she developed to calm and quiet herself. Her "Squeeze Machine," modeled after a cattle chute, applies firm pressure to the sides of the person's body, with the degree of pressure controlled by the person using it. Temple Grandin obtained a sense of relief and relaxation as well as pleasurable tactile stimulation when she was in this machine; and now, as she approaches age sixty, she still uses it at times.

Five-year-old Kenneth, described at the beginning of chapter 1, was standing on his head when I met him. It was his favorite position, his mother told me, one that he kept going back to as often as he was allowed. And, she added, he seemed to be more responsive after one of his head-standing periods. Other children with autism seem to crave movements like whirling or being swung around; and being allowed to jump on a mini-trampoline is rewarding enough to serve as a reinforcer in some behavioral programs.

The tactile defensiveness of many young children with autism will always remain clear in the minds of their parents: infants who arch their backs and cry in response to parents' attempts to hold them or who exhibit an aversion to being hugged or kissed or even touched. "Did you ever hear of a kid who didn't like piggyback?" William Christopher had asked plaintively, with his mind's eye on his own son. Even the refusal of some autistic children to keep their clothes on may be a defensive response to their sensitivity to certain textures, as some adults with autism explain. Something is amiss here, sensory integration theory would indicate, some dysfunction in the proprioceptive, vestibular, and/or tactile systems.

The proprioceptive system receives sensory information from our own bodies, specifically from the muscles and joints involved in movement. The vestibular system is responsive to gravity and to head movements, and it plays a role in awareness of body position, movement in space, and balance. According to sensory integration theory, when information from the vestibular, proprioceptive, and tactile systems is not integrated, the outcome is poor body awareness, attention, and motor planning as well as other developmental problems. Sensory integration therapy addresses this dysfunction through sensory stimulation and sensory motor challenges in activity contexts that are designed to elicit adaptive behavior. Deep pressure, massage, vibration, and play equipment like scooter boards, inclines, tunnels, swings, and sit-in toys that spin or rock are all commonly involved in sensory integration therapy with young children.

Sensory integration therapy is not meant to be the only therapy that a child with autism receives. It is often integrated into an educational treatment program or is adjunctive to it; parents of preschool children often arrange for this treatment along with speech services. Is this a waste of time? "Research indicates that the intervention [sensory integration therapy] does not help individuals function better" (Smith, Mruzek, and Mozingo 2005, 338). Or are the parents who have found this a helpful facilitative approach correct? Clearly, more good research on this subject is needed. Sensory integration therapy may not benefit most children with autism, but if I were a mother of an autistic child who appeared to have poor body awareness and coordination, who displayed tactile defensiveness, or who was extremely fearful of activities that provided sensory motor challenges, I would certainly want my child to have sensory integration therapy. I would try very hard, however, to ensure that this therapy did *not* cut into the intensity of my child's educational treatment.

"Breaking the Silence" was the title of an article in the August 1992 issue of *Teacher Magazine*. "Keyboard Helps Autistic Youths Find Their Voices, Advocates Say" was the name of another, in the June 11, 1992, issue of *Education Week*. In 1991 and 1992 facilitated communication was touted by the popular media as a miraculous way of opening up new worlds of possibility for people with autism. Article after article reported stories of children previously considered severely retarded who were typing meaningful and, in some cases, sophisticated ideas. This story, which appeared in the *New York Times Magazine,* was typical:

> At the Donald R. Ray Middle School in Baldwinsville, N. Y., 14-year-old Lucy Harrison seems eager to spend her speech-therapy session talking to a reporter. Although from time to time she says "yes" aloud, she converses primarily by typing with her left index finger on a small black portable typewriter. Her speech therapist, Kate Walsh, sits beside her, with her right hand gently supporting Lucy's forearm halfway between the elbow and wrist, her thumb resting on top and her four fingers underneath the arm, as though ready to catch it. Lucy rapidly taps out sentences, ignoring typographical errors in her haste.
>   As recently as 1989, Lucy was working at a first-grade level in a special-education classroom. This year, she was taking science, language arts and health in regular seventh-grade classes. Her most recent IQ tests place her in the high normal range, a leap of about 60 points, because she can now show her true abilities during testing. Without facilitation, Lucy types, "I would be helpless once again and it would be like a naked death." (Makarushka 1991, 70)

Yet by the mid 1990s the picture had changed sharply. What had been accepted as the unrecognized ability of children with autism was increasingly viewed as the communication of adult facilitators. Facilitated communication (FC) had undoubtedly become the most controversial intervention approach used with autistic individuals, and probably one of the most reviled. The tenor of articles and activities related to this intervention shifted dramatically. It was referred to as "antiscience" in the September 1995 issue of the prestigious journal *American Psychologist*. "A request for information about facilitated communication" was the subject of a January 30, 1996, joint memorandum from an assistant secretary in the U.S. Department of Education and a commissioner in the Department of Health and Human Services. The weight of influential institutions increasingly backed the antagonists of FC who cried "fraud." Charges of charlatanism were hurled at the professionals promoting or implementing facilitated communication. And almost everywhere today when facilitated communication is mentioned at all, it is referred to as a discredited treatment.

But facilitated communication had not suddenly appeared without any foundation; in fact, this approach has deep roots in observations of the behavior of children with autism and in early treatment strategies. More than thirty-five years ago, Dr. Mary Goodwin and her husband showed us that autistic children who don't communicate through speech may have unrecognized abilities. Mary and Campbell Goodwin were experienced pediatricians when they became interested in children with communication disorders. In their attempts to help such children they began using and testing the Edison Responsive Environment (E.R.E.), a cubicle containing a "talking typewriter" and programming device. The E.R.E. was made available for half-hour periods, one to five times a week, to each of sixty-five children diagnosed as having autism. Among the first children referred to the psychiatric clinic where the E.R.E. was located was a five-year-old boy with autistic behavior who had been excluded from kindergarten and was awaiting institutional placement. The Goodwins reported the following observations:

> We invited Robbie's mother to bring him to the center for a trial of the E.R.E. He was led to the door of the booth with the words "Here is a typewriter for you." When Robbie went home 15 minutes later, he had left behind him a full page of random typing interspersed with many words, "liquid," "final," "touch," "ivory," "downy," "chlorox". . . .
>
>   At later visits, he . . . wrote an original story paraphrased from "The Flintstones." (Goodwin and Goodwin 1969, 559–60)

Robbie was not the only child who demonstrated unexpected literacy on the typewriter. The Goodwins interpreted their findings to mean that the E.R.E. served to demonstrate abilities that go unrecognized because these children lack a means to express what they know. This is one of the central tenets of facilitated communication.

FC differs from what occurred in the Goodwins' project in that it involves physical support from an adult who serves as a "facilitator":

> Facilitated communication is a means by which many people with major speech difficulties point at letters on an alphabet board or typing device to convey their thoughts. It involves a facilitator who provides physical support to help stabilize the arm, to isolate the index finger if necessary, to pull back the arm after each selection, to remind the individual to maintain focus, and to offer emotional support and encouragement; the facilitator progressively phases out the physical support. (Biklen 1992, 243)

This "facilitation" is at the core of the controversy about facilitated communication. Why should such physical support be necessary? Professor Douglas Biklen of Syracuse University, the person who observed the use of facilitated communication in Australia and promoted it in the United States, proposed the idea that some autistic individuals have a problem with "praxis," that is, they have a neurologically based problem with expression that affects speaking and other ways of communicating. He pointed to a variety of observations and reports over the years to support this contention.

Normally developing infants are very good imitators, but children with autism spectrum disorders often have a deficit in the ability to imitate movement (Williams, Whiten, and Singh 2004). Why should this be? We don't really know, but one of the major explanations is that there may be an underlying motor dysfunction or dyspraxia in individuals with autism. Support for the idea of movement difficulties in autism comes also from anatomical studies. Postmortem examinations have identified abnormalities in the cerebellum, which is centrally involved in motor performance.

We have a long history of treating individuals with movement and communication disorders as mentally retarded. When institutions for the mentally retarded were dismantled in the mid to late 1970s, many of the people in these institutions were found to have cerebral palsy or multiple disabilities that interfered with the production of speech; but many of these individuals were not mentally retarded, even after years of neglect and deprivation. Today speech/language therapists routinely work on augmentative and alternative communication with children who have neuromotor disorders that interfere with the acquisition of speech. The use of augmentative and alternative communication, which may involve picture cards and boards, sign language, computers, and electronic devices with programming features as well as voice or print output, is a widely accepted strategy. It draws on the principle of making accommodations to meet the needs of individuals who cannot communicate in typical ways.

Facilitated communication may be considered a form of augmentative and alternative communication designed to accommodate the needs of individuals who are autistic (or otherwise disabled) and have dyspraxia. The terms "praxis," "dyspraxia," and "apraxia" are an integral part of the professional vocabulary of the field of occupational therapy. "Dyspraxia" refers to developmental disorders of motor planning that cause the child to have difficulty initiating and carrying out nonhabitual motor actions. If we accept the idea that autism reflects a neurological dysfunction or difference that may affect the production of speech and other forms of expression, it seems to make sense that some of these children may need special supports to facilitate writing and typing as well as speech. But FC has an inherent danger that is less likely to plague other types of augmentative and alternative communication—namely, that the facilitator's continuing physical support may result in a product representing the facilitator's ideas rather than those of the child or adult being assisted. This hazard and the situations it created explain why FC came to be widely viewed as a misguided and ineffective method or even as a hoax.

When I first learned of the work of Rosemary Crossley at the DEAL Communication Centre in Melbourne, Australia, I was quite excited. The approach she had developed in working with people who had cerebral palsy and was now also using with some autistic individuals appeared to confirm the combination of hope, fantasy, and wish of many parents and teachers that some children with autism knew more than they could show. A few months after Douglas Biklen began offering training in FC, I attended a workshop in New York City given by a special education teacher who had been trained at Syracuse University and had been using FC with her students. I came away from that workshop very uneasy. The workshop leader was highly enthusiastic about FC. Too enthusiastic? I asked myself. Facilitated communication was the answer in the air, and almost everyone seemed to be jumping on the bandwagon. FC had revived the concept of autism as a shell or cage that prevented the person inside from showing his or her true capabilities.

Two factors played critical roles in turning opinion virulently against facilitated communication: multiple accusations of sexual abuse, usually against family members; and conclusions from studies using conventional research designs that identified facilitators as the source of the messages being produced in almost all instances. Sexual abuse is often difficult to confirm; the testimony of the abused individual may be the only evidence available. When awareness of the possibility of facilitator influence became widespread, public and professional opinion sided strongly with the accused families. Given the uncertainty of the situation, this outcome is easy to understand: most of the accusations were undoubtedly false and quite damaging to families. And yet the case of Darla (Brantlinger, Klein, and Guskin 1994), a fifteen-year-old nonverbal woman with autism who was made pregnant by her fourteen-year-old brother in an apparently well-functioning family, illustrates the fact that unlikely events do occur in the lives of individuals with autism. The high rate of abuse, both physical and sexual, of individuals with disabilities has been documented for well over a decade.

What even the most ardent promoters of FC did not dispute was that in many cases facilitators inadvertently determined the content of the typed communications. The issue that remained was whether facilitator influence on content was so endemic to FC that it accounted for virtually all the unexpected findings of literacy in individuals with autism. Almost all research studies have answered that question with a "yes" (Jacobson, Foxx, and Mulick 2005). Proponents of FC point out that some individuals with autism can communicate independently after working with FC for some time. However, the number of persons with autism who have used FC and now type independently while continuing to demonstrate the same level of literacy and sophisticated thinking appears to be extremely small.

Where does that leave us? Is facilitated communication totally without value? Is it harmful? One type of harm that FC may have caused was to stop teachers and family members from trying to develop literacy skills in their students or children because FC led them to believe falsely that these individuals already had such skills. Yet withdrawing access to FC altogether, which is what has occurred, is a draconian measure. It cuts off a channel of expression for those individuals with autism, however small their number, who have complex ideas they can't otherwise express; and it removes a potentially valuable teaching tool for helping nonverbal individuals with autism acquire literacy, including skill in written communication. Chapter 3 introduced Morton Ann Gernsbacher's son, who at age nine was a student in a virtual high school. He developed his skill in computer learning and communication with instruction and practice starting as a toddler, and he has been typing independently for years. But when he is overwhelmed or upset, his mother reports, he still needs a supportive hand on his shoulder in order to get started on his computer.

Tito Mukhoppadhyay is an adolescent with autism who garnered much attention after he and his mother arrived in the United States from India with the sponsorship of Cure Autism Now (CAN). Tito cannot communicate his ideas through speech; his speech is virtually unintelligible. He has an extremely high level of stereotyped movements that include hand flapping and head swiveling. He can't look at you and listen to what you are saying at the same time. He appears severely autistic, but he also writes poetry. Tito was not a participant in a facilitated communication program, but he learned to write and to type on a computer after years of being read to, instructed, and physically prompted by his mother. Without his mother's physical guidance of his hands or support at his shoulder, he was not able to initiate the necessary movements to write. Tito still sometimes writes with a pencil but also types independently. He is an example of a person with autism whose outer appearance belies his abilities. He was very fortunate to have a mother who was able and willing to devote herself entirely to him and who sensed what assistance he needed. Tito is a person with autism who might not have had a communication channel if he had not had a mother who used her own version of facilitated communication as a teaching tool.

Rather than totally dismissing FC as a destructive hoax, we should try to figure out how it can be used beneficially for different individuals—as a teaching/learning mode first and then as a means of expression later on for some, being careful to avoid the pitfalls of the past. The concept of a cognitively competent, literate individual trapped inside a facade of autism is undoubtedly relevant to far fewer individuals than the initial reports on FC made it appear; but given the great diversity of the autistic population, why can't we consider the idea that some individuals with autism may know much more than they can communicate, while others may know very little more than the fragments they show us? Should we be in the business of cutting off access to any approach that might be useful to some people with autism who have not been able to establish verbal communication and appear to be dyspraxic, because that approach does not hold the whole answer we had hoped for? Or should we acknowledge that FC is an approach that was implemented in a naïve and misguided way, motivated by hope and dreams, with sometimes harmful effects; without rejecting the idea that it might hold the possibility of real communication for some individuals failed by other methods?

As long as there are children with autism spectrum disorders who are not developing in the typical way for reasons unknown to us, and as long as there is no known cure or highly effective treatment that can help all of them function in ways close to what is viewed as typical and desirable, there will be alternative treatments and procedures designed to achieve this goal. Sometimes children with autism will be helped by these interventions, and sometimes they won't be. We can inform parents about the plausibility of treatments and about the quality and quantity of evidence that supports or doesn't support these approaches. We can alert parents to potential treatment dangers and present advice on how to minimize risks. What we can't do is stop parents from having a dream and trying to make it come true—nor should we.

PART THREE

Looking for Cures,
Recovery, and Better Lives

9 Recovery?

"Autism" is spoken of by some people as a jigsaw with a missing piece. I experienced my own "autism" as one bucket with several different jigsaws in it, all jumbled together and all missing a few pieces each but with a few extra pieces that didn't belong to any of these jigsaws. From there, I had to work out which pieces were missing and which ones weren't supposed to be in my bucket at all.

(Williams 1996, 1)

One evening I was sitting in the rear of an almost empty bus when I noticed a young man walking toward the back of the bus and casually observed him. Something about him was familiar, I suddenly realized. When he sat on a seat adjacent to mine, I was sure. "Are you Victor W.?" I asked. "Who are you? How do you know me?" he replied.

Victor had been a student in my class seventeen years earlier. He was ten years old the last time I'd seen him. How did I recognize him? What first made him appear familiar was his walk, sometimes referred to as toe walking. It was less pronounced than when he was a child but still noticeable. The second memory trigger was his partial smile, not a communicative smile, not meant for anyone else. What made me sure it was Victor, the same Victor I described in chapter 6, was the mouth movements — tiny, rudimentary word formations that accompanied his thinking.

When Victor left my class and the treatment center in which it was located, he went to a small private school. We had all worked hard to help him make that transition. Now, after some initial discomfort at my mention of how I knew him, Victor joyfully told me about his adult life. He was a doctoral student in an area of science. I remembered that his parents had wanted him to be a doctor and that the head of the treatment team had referred to this wish as evidence of the father's tenuous acceptance of Victor's condition. He had, in fact, tried to get into medical school, Victor told me, but wasn't accepted. He was married now, and he told me about his wife's work. As his stop approached, Victor gave me a warm goodbye and departed. We had talked for almost twenty minutes.

I was amazed and elated over this encounter. I remembered Victor as he was when he entered my class after five years of treatment. He had an excellent memory and a large store of information, but his thinking was concrete and rigid, and any unanticipated event could throw him into a frenzy. For a year we worked on abstracting and generalizing, adapting and coping, self-monitoring and self-control. I felt cautiously optimistic that he would succeed in his regular education class, which contained only eight students because the school had just opened, but never did I anticipate that someday he would become a PhD candidate. As soon as I arrived home that evening, I checked the telephone directory. His name was there, and just seeing it there, the concreteness and certainty of it, increased my elation, just as concreteness and certainty had made Victor feel secure many years earlier.

A year or two later, I saw a notice in a university newsletter under the heading "Alumni News." It was about Victor W., Ph.D., and gave his workplace and title—along with the name of an article he had written that had just been published in a journal. A number of years have passed since my chance meeting with Victor, but for years I saw his name listed in that same newsletter under alumni donors to the university fund. Had Victor recovered? Possibly. It depends on what is meant by recovery.

That word "recovery," the rallying cry of parents of young children with autism who believe in Lovaas and Catherine Maurice, a word otherwise unheard in relation to autism, is a word with an implied promise: normalcy. Your child can be normal. How did this word enter the dictionary of autism when most highly regarded professionals viewed autism as a lifelong disorder?

Everyone wants children with autism to overcome its devastating effects—the fear and pain, the inability to communicate, the areas of developmental arrest, and the isolation, self-abuse, and destructiveness that are sometimes part of the picture. In 1996 and 1997, when I wrote the first edition of this book, "recovery" was the most contentious issue in the field of autism, fueled by the reports of Ivar Lovaas. Today both written references to autism as a lifelong disorder and claims of "recovery" from programs using applied behavior analysis are generally more muted. This no longer constitutes the central focus of attention, which has shifted to causes, prevention, and treatments that might afford a life of better options and greater possibilities. But for parents recovery is still the ever-present hope, and it is parents who are using multiple intervention strategies, including biomedical treatment, who are claiming recovery most often. Bernard Rimland is probably the most notable professional (and a parent as well) who is supporting parental claims of recovery today. In the proceedings of the 2005 DAN! conference he writes: "The number of recoveries is increasing every day. Soon it will be tens of thousands" (Autism Research Institute 2005); and through the institute that he directs he disseminates a DVD entitled "Recovered Autistic Children" (Autism Research Institute 2004).

There have always been claims that children with autism have overcome that condition and have begun to function normally, but until Lovaas reported his treatment outcomes in 1987 these were isolated claims about a tiny percentage of individuals with autism. There are various possible meanings for the claim of recovery. Does recovery mean that possible neurobiological factors underlying autism—differences in the structure or functioning of the brain, for example—have been eliminated? Or does it mean that while these neurobiological differences still exist, the behavioral differences that reflected them have been reduced so significantly that the individual no longer meets the criteria for autism or any other developmental disability, although he or she continues to exhibit odd behavior and unusual adaptive strategies? Or does it mean that the individual's functioning is no longer distinguishable from what is considered typical or normal?

No one claims to have eliminated the neurobiological factors that may give rise to autism, although it is conceivable that intensive early learn-ing experiences might cause alterations in the neurological system. Since we don't thoroughly understand what factors underlie autism, we can't assess changes in them. This takes us to the second and third possible definitions of recovery. We can view these definitions in relation to Temple Grandin. Some people, impressed with her PhD, work success, writing, and presentations, might think of Temple as recovered, but she considers herself a person with autism. She has developed her own per-sonal catalog of strategies to handle common situations that she finds particularly difficult, so that for the most part she manages her life quite well. Yet she clearly differs from most people in the way she has to deal with such basic functions as learning, thinking, and remembering; she still has unusual difficulty coping with certain types of social interac-tions; and she has only relatively recently, in middle age, begun to have what most people would consider real friendships.

After the publication of her 1995 book, Temple participated in book signings. One such event took place at a meeting of a local chapter of the Autism Society of America, where she was to make a presentation. When I entered the auditorium I saw Temple standing with her back to the wall near a table stacked with copies of her book. At the other side was a pub-lisher's representative. Temple spoke neither to him nor to any of the peo-ple who asked for her signature. When I brought my copy to her, I tried to begin a conversation, pointing out that I had purchased her book ear-lier and had read it thoroughly, as she could see from the slips of paper sticking out of it at various places. There was no response from Temple. She silently signed her name, nothing more. Later, during her animated and impressive presentation, she mentioned that she never wrote any-thing but her name in her books because she didn't know what else to write. In *An Anthropologist on Mars*, Oliver Sacks has this to say about the question of recovery in relation to Temple Grandin: "'Normality' had been revealed more and more, as we spoke, as a sort of front, or facade, for her, albeit a brave and often brilliant front, behind which she remained, in some ways, as far 'outside,' as unconnected, as ever" (1995, 275).

Catherine Maurice's children reached a point where they no longer met the criteria for autism, but were their difficulties in communication and social functioning eliminated, or did her children achieve generally normal outcomes by different routes? Are these difficulties totally gone or will differences—residuals or shadows of autism—show up later in their adolescence and adulthood? Before the question of recovery can be examined productively, an operational definition must be specified.

The mother of the university graduate mentioned in chapter 2 told the audience waiting to hear her son's presentation, "My son and I have both rediscovered his autism. He was diagnosed as autistic as a child. Then the label was removed, and we thought he used to be autistic; but now we know he is autistic." The term "recovered" doesn't fit her son well. There are a good number of adults with autism who look normal in many ways but who still feel different and still have difficulty dealing with some basic aspects of everyday life.

Since the controversy over the word "recovery" stemmed primarily from the claims of Lovaas, let's look at how he defined this term. In his 1987 article "Behavioral Treatment and Normal Educational and Intellectual Functioning in Young Autistic Children"—which caught the attention of the academic world—Lovaas reported that nine out of nineteen children who participated in his intensive behavioral treatment program had achieved normal functioning by age seven. He used the term "recovered" a couple of times in that article to refer to these nine children. By normal functioning, Lovaas meant having an IQ in the average range, being maintained in regular education classes, and being promoted from grade to grade. He did acknowledge, however, that some children can meet this definition of normal functioning and still have residual deficits that may become obvious only as a child gets older, much like the university graduate who lost his autism label in childhood only to reclaim it later. But the recovery claims that Lovaas made go beyond the operational definition used in 1987. In a film showing five boys who had been part of his Young Autism Project, three of whom were identified as having recovered, Lovaas essentially challenged the viewer to distinguish two of these adolescents from their friends in the film. Indeed, on the basis of the brief film footage provided, I could not make this discrimination.

The follow-up study reported in 1993 (McEachin, Smith, and Lovaas) added other measures to assess whether the children considered to have normal functioning had residual deficits—the Vineland Adaptive Behavior Scales, the Personality Inventory for Children, and a clinical interview. Lovaas and his associates concluded that eight of the nine children did not have residual deficits, but this conclusion was questioned by many other professionals, who counseled caution in accepting the follow-up data as sufficient proof of completely normal functioning or recovery. Nonetheless, these adolescents appeared to have achieved essentially normal functioning.

What is the future for individuals with autism? How do most children with autism turn out or fare as adults? This is the broader context into which questions about recovery should be placed. The answer to the question of outcomes can best be obtained from follow-up studies of children with autism who have reached adolescence or adulthood. An analysis of eight early follow-up studies found a common pattern: from 5–17 percent of autistic children had good outcomes, while 61–74 percent had poor or very poor outcomes, and the remainder had fair outcomes (Lotter 1978). The definition of "good outcome" used in this analysis was normal or near-normal social life along with satisfactory functioning at school or work. This definition is not equivalent to recovery, but it would include instances of recovery.

Perhaps the most interesting of the early follow-up studies are those done by Leo Kanner, which were reported in his 1973 book *Childhood Psychosis: Initial Studies and New Insights.* Twenty-eight years after the appearance of his groundbreaking 1943 article, which introduced the concept of "autistic disturbances," he conducted a follow-up study of eight of the eleven children described in that publication. Kanner found that two of them had good outcomes, and one of these two had achieved very close to normal functioning. This individual was a college graduate who did well at his job as a bank teller. He also belonged to a variety of organizations including a local Kiwanis club, where he had served a term as president. Even so, his mother, while very proud of his accomplishments, described him as not completely normal; he did not express his inner feelings, rarely participated in social conversation, and displayed little initiative (Kanner 1973).

Another study reexamined forty-two children Kanner had diagnosed as having autism. Only one could be considered to have achieved normal functioning. A third follow-up report on autistic children seen at Johns Hopkins Hospital, where Kanner was based, involved ninety-six children. This study identified nine individuals with good outcomes, with the criteria for a good outcome being employability, absence of obvious behavior problems, and satisfactory social relationships. Of these nine, four had college degrees, two were attending college, and three were employed full time. None of the nine had married, but five of them lived independently, and several were dating.

None of the studies just described reported anything like the percentage of children apparently achieving normal functioning in the Lovaas program, but treatment was not a major variable in any of these studies, and intensive treatment of any kind was rarely available. However, in the late 1960s Kanner conducted a follow-up study of children who had been involved in an intensive treatment program at the Linwood Children's Center in Maryland. Founded by a teacher, Linwood was a center specifically for children considered psychotic, a good many of whom met Kanner's definition of autism. The center's approach stressed acceptance of the children and their behavior as well as expansion of that behavior into more varied and functional activities. The treatment framework was developmental/psychodynamic. Kanner concluded that at least six of the fifteen autistic children he studied had achieved either full recovery or close to normal functioning. They did well in mainstream educational programs, had friends, and engaged in a variety of age-appropriate activities such as sports. The center's rate of normal or close to normal outcomes was considerably higher than the rate reported in other studies, and not much less than the recovery rate reported by Lovaas. This finding underscores the value of intensive educational treatment and supports the idea that interventions that differ significantly from the behavioral approach used by Lovaas and his followers can result in very good outcomes for some children with autism.

A somewhat more recent study conducted in Toronto (Szatmari et al. 1989) focused on sixteen adults who had been treated at a center for autistic children under the age of six and who had IQs above 65 at the time they were in treatment at that center. The outcomes for this group were considerably better than outcomes reported in other studies that included children with lower IQs. Four of the adults would have been considered normal by most people unfamiliar with their childhood functioning. Thus, 25 percent of these adults seemed to have achieved essentially normal functioning. Although the twelve other adults continued to have problems in functioning, several had higher education degrees, and three held jobs in the community. This study did not focus on the effects of treatment, but it may well be that the treatment all these individuals received during early childhood contributed to their better than expected outcomes.

A 1991 analysis of outcome studies (Gillberg) concluded that whereas the vast majority of children with autism remain severely socially restricted in adulthood, a very small number of such children appear to "grow out of autism" and have extremely good outcomes. As older adolescents and adults they are indistinguishable or almost indistinguishable from nondisabled people. This conclusion breeds both hope and fear in parents and other caring adults—hope that their child will be one of those who becomes indistinguishable from nondisabled individuals, and fear that their child may be one of the larger proportion of children with autism who will remain severely restricted in later life.

A large Swedish follow-up study of individuals born between 1962 and 1984 who were diagnosed with autism did not identify any adults with good outcomes (Billstedt, Gillberg, and Gillberg 2005). One of the 108 individuals no longer met criteria for an autism spectrum disorder but nonetheless did not do well, and 57 percent of the sample had very poor outcomes. These results probably reflect underidentification of children with better functioning, older age at identification and at the start of intervention, and less well developed intervention systems for this population during those years. Certainly, the data from this study contrast sharply with outcomes reported by programs in the United States in recent years.

Phillip Strain reported on the outcomes of the first six children to complete LEAP, a preschool program described in chapter 6 (Strain and Hoyson 2000). At age ten, none of the children met criteria for autism; their noncompliant behavior with mothers had been largely eliminated; their positive social interaction levels were similar to those of their typical peers; five of the six had been in mainstream class placements without special education services since leaving LEAP; and the mean IQ of this group was 101. Were five of these children "recovered"? They certainly had achieved very good outcomes, but Strain makes no claim of recovery; nor does he provide enough individual data to consider this question closely.

What an analysis of follow-up studies does not give us is a blueprint for increasing the number of children who become indistinguishable from nondisabled people or almost so. During the past few years, earlier identification of children on the autism spectrum and changes in federal education law have combined to make treatment of two- and three-year-old children with autism much more common, and many of these children receive services specifically designed for this population. This change can be expected to lead to an increase in the percentage of children with autism who achieve very good outcomes.

Anecdotal reports and case studies of recovery from autism have appeared in the literature from time to time over many years. They tell us a different part of the story of recovery. Perhaps the best publicized case of recovery is that of Raun Kaufman, whose father, Barry, has told this story many times in different forms. The story became well known through Barry Kaufman's 1976 book *Son Rise* and a 1979 television movie based on this book. A revised edition containing an update and additional case studies was published in 1994 under the title *Son Rise: The Miracle Continues*.

Even before their son's diagnosis, the Kaufmans thought "autism" and began a search for answers. They found none that satisfied them—not from Ivar Lovaas or Bernard Rimland or Bruno Bettelheim—and day by day they saw their infant son slipping away from them. Their answer? They would create their own path, their own way of accepting and reaching their gentle but distant child. They observed him intensively, looking for clues to ways of connecting and communicating with him. They joined him in his spinning and rocking rituals, trying to break into his world. His environment was simplified, and all his waking hours were spent with a parent or other caregiver, with about six hours a day of structured or semi-structured activities. Raun was seventeen months old when the program began. A formal evaluation when he was twenty months old showed an autistic child whose language and social development were like those of an infant of about eight months. The next evaluation, at twenty-four months, showed age-appropriate developmental levels in all areas.

Shortly after his first book appeared, I invited Barry Kaufman to address the course I had just introduced into the master's degree program in special education at Hunter College, titled Working with Parents of Young Handicapped Children. He came. His son was five at that time and was in nursery school. In some ways Raun was functioning above his age level, Kaufman told my students, but some unusual behavior was still present. He was very touch-oriented, for example, and if he saw a baby in a carriage, he might go up to it and stroke its face, an action not usually viewed in a favorable light by the infant's parents. Kaufman had no doubt, however, that his son would do fine in school and elsewhere.

About twelve years later I received some promotional material for the Option Institute that Barry Kaufman and his wife, Samahria (Suzi in his first book), had established in Sheffield, Massachusetts, to teach their philosophy and approach to other families and professionals. A brochure described Raun as a ninth grader attending public school who had been a straight A student for several years, who had an IQ of 150, who was highly gregarious, and who had no residual signs of autism. In 1994 two additional pieces of information about Raun appeared in print. An article in the *New York Teacher*, the newsletter of the state teachers' union, described Raun as a senior at an Ivy League college majoring in biomedical ethics; and Raun himself, in the foreword to his father's revised book, informed us that he was on his college's debating team, loved Stephen King novels, wrote science fiction stories, had a girlfriend, drove a car, was studying ballroom dancing, and was a member of a fraternity. Recovered? It certainly seemed so.

Several years after that I watched and listened to Raun at a meeting where he talked about the treatment center that his parents had established and in which he now worked. His performance appeared both sincere and polished. Had I not known his history I would not have suspected that he had ever been diagnosed with autism. Does that confirm "recovery"? Not necessarily, but it does confirm that excellent outcomes with essentially normal functioning are possible for some individuals who have not had ABA treatment.

Several years ago I received a package at my college office. It was a book manuscript written by a father about his daughter, who was then five and a half, and her "successful struggle against autism." I called this father and talked to him about his daughter and the intervention process that he and his wife used. They had learned the approach at the Option Institute. For four years after that I heard nothing further about the child or the book, which the father had wanted to publish, so I called him again. The manuscript had not been published, he reported; he had decided that he didn't want his daughter to be known as the girl who had been autistic. She was now functioning like other children in all ways, he told me, except that she was two years behind in her development because of the time she had lost to autism. At age six she had entered a pre-kindergarten class instead of the first grade. Since then she had been progressing at the usual rate and was doing well in school. She had friends, was very well liked, and participated in neighborhood activities.

How had this been achieved? I asked this father. By twelve hours of work, day in and day out, for four years, with the help of many volunteers, he replied. The treatment program had taken some time to begin working, but after two years his daughter was almost out of her autism; in four years there were no traces of autism left, he stated. Yes, the Option Institute did charge a lot of money for the Son-Rise program, the father agreed, but it was worth it. Before they visited the Option Institute they had been at their wit's end, what with their daughter's tantrums, her attacks on them, and the injuries she inflicted on herself. The Son-Rise program was certainly worth the money, this father told me, because it helped them rescue their child from autism and saved their family.

The Son-Rise model generated tremendous controversy in the 1990s, largely because it broke all the rules: it wasn't developed by professionals, wasn't directed by someone with professional credentials in autism, described its methods only in very broad terms, and didn't collect or report outcome data in ways considered acceptable by the professional community. This model apparently led to an excellent outcome for Raun Kaufman and a few other children, but what about the many others whose families used it? According to Barry Kaufman, the Son-Rise approach has "facilitated deep-seated and lasting change in hundreds of children and their families" (1994, 245). Unfortunately, he did not define "deep-seated change" in terms of specific outcomes; therefore, we have no idea of how many of these hundreds of children achieved anything approaching typical functioning or even moderately good outcomes. "Deep-seated and lasting change in children and families" can mean that parents have come to accept their child's autism and its implications instead of being in a constant state of turmoil and conflict about it, as one mother who used this approach and whose daughter had made little progress toward more typical behavior reported to me.

Some individuals with autism clearly do achieve near-normal functioning. They graduate from college, have better than average IQs, and participate in activities in the community; but they may have few if any close friends, may have difficulty with adult love relationships, often have trouble obtaining and maintaining jobs commensurate with their education and ability, and feel different from "typicals" in significant ways. Drew Johnson is one of the successes of Ivar Lovaas's Young Autism Project. During his second year of college Drew wrote the afterword in his mother's book about his recovery. At one point he states:

> I do have trouble expressing my feelings to others. The main reason I believe is that I have a linear thought process. I don't know why I think like this because my mom, brother, and sister are very emotional. I do express my emotions in extreme cases. For example, when a family member dies or when one of my friends gets screwed. There is a good side, however. The fact that I am not very emotional helps me in every decision I have to make. (Johnson and Crowder 1994, 182)

Personality difference or residue of autism or residue shading into personality?

The studies and stories presented in this chapter focus on individuals who were diagnosed with autism. Asperger syndrome was not yet a recognized label when most of these children were diagnosed, but what of the children who were identified as having Asperger syndrome in early childhood? Have they "recovered" or achieved typical functioning? A very successful businessman of twenty-seven has not "recovered" from Asperger syndrome, although he appears to function normally. He explains that he has managed to be successful both because of some of his special characteristics and in spite of them. He is excellent at using visualization to identify patterns in apparently random data, a skill that he attributes to his Asperger syndrome; and he has consciously and intensively focused on learning how people are likely to respond. While he appears "normal" on the surface, after about an hour of "seemingly informal conversation with people" he is completely exhausted (Jacobs 2003, 84–85).

The title of Liane Willey's first book is *Pretending to Be Normal*, which is something that she tried to do for most of her life. To some extent she succeeded, but in other ways she did not. About "recovery" she writes:

> As most of my AS traits continue to fade away, I have noticed the most tenacious of the lot . . . popping up here and there . . . teasing me from the thought that I will ever be anyone else's normal. Try as I might to catch and contain them, these are the qualities I will never lose. (Willey 1999, 77)

The appearance of typicality is sometimes achieved by special strategies. Liane Willey has lists of how to act. Included on her list are items pertaining to her behavior with her husband—"hold Tom's hand for five minutes every day" and "hug Tom three times today" (1999, 84). She has learned that these demonstrations of affection are important to good relationships with a spouse, but she has to program them; they don't come naturally to her. Liane Willey tells us that she has found a mostly comfortable place in life for herself somewhere between neurologically typical and Asperger syndrome.

In his book *Beyond the Wall* (2003) Stephen Shore indicates that he challenged the walls that kept him locked in the castle of autism and was cleared for takeoff (his metaphors), but he does not claim recovery. He recognizes residuals of his Asperger syndrome, his difficulty with facial recognition being one example.

During the past ten or so years, and particularly during the more recent of those years, adults with milder versions of autism spectrum disorders have become much more visible. This undoubtedly reflects the increase in the number of individuals identified as having Asperger syndrome, more open communication about autism spectrum disorders, and the achievement of better treatment outcomes. Networks of adults with autism spectrum disorders have sprung up, and a rather unique culture has developed. Members communicate through their computers and at meetings or retreats. How is this culture different? Where else could you find badges color-coded to indicate that the wearer does not want to be spoken to at all or wants to be spoken to only by friends? Where else would you see a button reading "I survived behavior modification," or a shirt that reads "Cure all neurotypicals, but don't cure me" (Paradiz 2002, 138–39)? Where else would you hear a conversation like the one that follows?

> Stephen looks at me, smiling. "That's fairly asparagus of you."
> "What?"
> "Asparagus. That's what some of us Aspies call ourselves. Asperger's, asparagus. Are you sure you're not an asparagus?" (Adams 2005, 277)

Parents have mixed feelings about this. On the one hand, parents of young children with severe impairments are gladdened by the abilities of these individuals. On the other hand, some parents, probably many of those with young children, don't accept the idea that their child may continue to have characteristics of autism spectrum disorders and may later claim membership in an autism culture.

Some parents and many professionals decry references to "recovery" or any other term that might imply that autism can be cured. They feel that such references are misleading and cruel, that they fuel hopes that will not be realized. Yes, it is true that there is no known cure for autism, and many families will be disappointed when the treatments that reportedly produced individuals like Raun Kaufman or the Maurice children don't result in similar outcomes for their son or daughter. We need to be very careful about making any claims that will mislead parents, but we also need to take care not to wipe out their hopes. We need stories of triumph, and we need other stories to show that even if recovery is not possible, individuals with autism are leading better lives—lives that have more satisfactions—than was ever possible in the past.

"Recovery from autism is different from recovery from everything else, and one can split hairs endlessly," Christina Adams writes (2005, 309). "If Jonah has some ADHD traits, some social weaknesses . . . if he has to take medicine and be on a diet to stay healthy, is that recovery?" she asks about her son, who no longer meets criteria for autism, PDD-NOS. or Asperger syndrome. Lynn Hamilton says this about the question of her son's recovery:

> Is Ryan recovered? That depends on the eye of the beholder. Many parents can't distinguish Ryan from typical children, but we know residual symptoms still need to be addressed. We also believe that Ryan has some underlying biomedical issues that need to be identified and dealt with in the coming years. . . . What has happened over these past four years is that Ryan is no longer confined by his autism. His life has been reclaimed, and he is enjoying it to the fullest. (Hamilton 2000, 305)

An accumulation of evidence collected over more than thirty years from multiple sources shows that some individuals with autism do go on to enjoy an essentially normal life or something very close to it. Such individuals have had varying life experiences that are not associated with only one particular type of treatment. It is also clear that other individuals with autism have achieved lives that appear normal on casual viewing but, on closer scrutiny, are not. "Jean-Paul is not 'cured.' He . . . still has problems related to his autism," writes the mother of this man who has two master's degrees, in the introduction to a newsletter article by her son (Bovee 1995, 6). This is the same Jean-Paul who stated during a presentation that he could engage in great conversation or eye contact, but not both at the same time.

A parent asked, What if my son remains autistic? What will we do? The best you can—with your love, your skills, and all the resources you can marshal—to help him achieve as independent and joyful a life as is possible for him.

10 Moving toward Better Answers

New technologies in gene research can allow scientists to better understand the role genes play in the development of autism, and eventually lead to better treatments.

(National Institute of Mental Health 2005)

More than forty years have passed since I was a teacher of Nellie, Sean, and other children with autism. If these children had been born after 1995 instead of before 1965, could I or others have helped them more? Could they have more easily come to understand the world around them and learned better ways to communicate their needs and ideas to others? Could Nellie's hand biting have been avoided? Could Sean have reached a point where head banging was only a thing of the past? Could they have gone to schools and been in classes with other children from their neighborhoods? It's impossible to answer these questions with any certainty, but Nellie and Sean would have a much better chance of reaching these markers of typicality today.

Why is this true? What has changed? Recognition of autism has changed. It's no longer a condition that's ignored or brushed aside until a child reaches age four or five. Children with autism are increasingly being diagnosed at two years of age or younger. Society's attitude toward individuals with severe disabilities, including autism, has changed. We no longer believe that people who are very different in some ways need to be shut off from the world of "typicals." Children with autism are not sent to institutions, as Sean was, although a very small number reside in treatment centers for varying lengths of time. The educational service picture has changed. It's no longer necessary to fight for education for a child with autism or wait until that child is five or six before he or she can go to school. Early intervention services are now being provided to an increasing number of two-year-olds. Today children who go to special schools usually do so because their parents believe that they will receive more help there, not because no other options are available. And no teacher today is expected to be the sole adult in a classroom with six to eight autistic students, as I was in the 1960s. How much more I could do for Nellie, I used to think, if only there were another adult in the classroom so that I could work with Nellie alone for chunks of time during the school day.

All of this is true, but it's no guarantee that Nellie and Sean would do well today, only that they would have a much better chance for a good life. We still don't know enough to help all the Nellies and Seans, and only a lucky few get the best of what we do know today about treating children with autism. Let's look at what we can do, need to do, if the Nellies and Seans of today are to have a better chance at a fuller life.

There are four major avenues for improving the lives of individuals with autism or eliminating autism from their lives altogether. The first is to identify the etiology of autism spectrum disorders and develop methods to correct the original deviation(s) or differences that lead to the behavioral syndrome called autism—in other words, to find a way to prevent or cure autism. Until this is possible, however, other avenues must be pursued. A second route to improving the lives of individuals with autism is to achieve a better understanding of the biological paths this disorder takes as it moves toward observable behavior—that is, to understand the systems it affects and how it affects them so that we can design more targeted and effective medical, pharmacological, perhaps dietary, and other possible treatments for individuals on the spectrum. The third route is to improve educational and behavioral treatment by finding ways to match intervention strategies to the particular characteristics and needs of individual children. The fourth avenue is to create greater equity in the provision of treatment by bringing publicly funded intervention services closer to the state of the art and closer to what families with abundant resources obtain for their children.

What we are searching for ultimately are answers at the biological level. Without understanding the biological substrate(s) of autism spectrum disorders, we grope about in semi-darkness. Still, this is an exciting time in biomedical research. Almost weekly, newspapers and magazines carry stories about breakthroughs in our understanding of how human biological systems operate and about the kinds of breakdowns in these systems that lead to various types of medical conditions and disorders in behavior.

It has been only a few years since serious funding and major research efforts began to be devoted to autism. The mid to late 1990s saw the beginning of this movement, with support coming from the National Institutes of Health (NIH) for the establishment of an international network of Collaborative Programs of Excellence in Autism. The Children's Health Act of 2000, achieved largely through the advocacy efforts of parent-organized groups, supplied additional momentum to this movement. That act directed NIH to expand, intensify, and coordinate its activities in regard to autism research. A direct outcome of this law was the establishment of a new autism research network—the Studies to Advance Autism Research and Treatment program. STAART centers conduct basic and clinical research into the cause, early identification, diagnosis, prevention, and treatment of autism, utilizing knowledge from the fields of genetics, developmental neurobiology, and psychopharmacology. The Children's Health Act of 2000 also directed that samples of genetic materials be made available for research. Such a program was established through the Human Genetics Initiative of NIH, and DNA samples, cell lines, and clinical data are now available to researchers. NIH has also joined forces with private foundations to support genetic research on autism.

While there has been a huge expansion of research on autism during the last few years, we still don't have the answers that are needed to break the code of autism. As this edition of *Targeting Autism* is being completed, advocacy activities in the autism community in support of the Combating Autism Act are escalating. This act would build on the provisions of the Children's Health Act and would authorize more federal funds to combat autism over a period of five years. It would also expand the network of centers of Excellence in Autism.

In the meantime, studies of the neuropathology of autism are producing valuable clues to differences in brain structure and function in individuals with autism spectrum disorders. No longer are researchers looking for one brain structure or region that is grossly abnormal. Instead, what is now envisioned are multiple areas with more subtle differences. One difference that has recently gained widespread recognition relates to brain size (Hazlett et al. 2005). While head circumference at birth is normal in children who later develop autism, by two years of age brain size is usually larger than normal. Increased brain size is not maintained after childhood. This phenomenon is not yet well understood.

Dr. Margaret Bauman of the Department of Pediatrics and Neurology at Massachusetts General Hospital has been studying the anatomy of the brain in autism for about two decades using autopsy material from children and young adults who died as a result of injury or illness. She has identified several differences in brain structure between individuals with autism and matched controls. The limbic system of the brain, believed to play a major role in emotion, is the seat of several of these differences. The amygdala, part of the limbic system sometimes referred to as the brain's "emotional computer," appears to mediate several responses—motivation, attention, and representation—involved in social orienting, joint attention, and recognition of the affective significance of stimuli. Bauman found that neurons in the amygdala of individuals with autism are smaller and more densely packed than those in people without autism, perhaps because the early pruning of neurons that normally takes place had not occurred. This could lead to curtailment of normal neuronal development. Such limbic system abnormalities might be involved in producing some of the core characteristics of autism.

Bauman has also identified abnormalities in the cerebellum, which is considered the coordinating center for movement and is thought to ensure optimal performance of voluntary motor acts. The cerebellum may also have a role in the modulation of sensory input, attention, emotion, and some aspects of language. Thus, abnormalities in the cerebellum may contribute to difficulties in sensory processing and motor planning as well as to other characteristics of autism (Bauman and Kemper 2005).

With autism now widely viewed as a disorder of neuronal organization, neuroimaging is increasingly being used to study individuals with this condition, and imaging research is beginning to produce important information about neural structures and mechanisms. Findings from studies using magnetic resonance imaging (MRI) provide some support for the anatomical differences in the cerebellum identified by Bauman. Eric Courchesne, who pioneered the use of magnetic resonance imaging, has argued that the cerebellum ensures optimal performance of several neural systems, for example, the sensory and attentional systems, to which it is functionally connected. Thus, cerebellar abnormality could place the young autistic child on a developmental pathway that Courchesne and his associates refer to as "misorganizing" (1994). Such a pathway would be consistent with the descriptions by autistic adults of their fragmented and confusing experiences in childhood.

The frontal lobes of the brain have been identified as critical to planning, impulse control, organized problem solving, and flexibility in thinking and acting, areas in which many individuals with autism spectrum disorders have difficulty. These processes are often referred to as executive functions. On neuropsychological tests designed to assess planning and flexibility in problem solving, children with autism and either normal or near-normal IQs perform significantly more poorly than nonautistic children of the same mental age. Moreover, frontal lobe damage in childhood is known to impair the ability to understand the viewpoints of others and to demonstrate appropriate empathy, characteristics often found in autistic persons. A number of neuroimaging studies have reported differences in frontal lobe activity between children with autism and typically developing children. This is an area of research that continues to be explored.

Neurochemicals are involved in multiple aspects of neural development, and abnormal brain chemistry has been identified in several conditions thought of as mental disorders. A number of studies have found abnormalities of the neurotransmitter serotonin in children and adults with autism. Research on differences between autistic and nonautistic children in regard to serotonin and other neurochemicals may lead to new and more effective treatments.

At present, no drug has been approved by the U.S. Food and Drug Administration specifically to treat autism. This area of treatment is still in its infancy (Steingard, Connor, and Au 2005). The drugs used with some individuals who have autism spectrum disorders act on selected behaviors found in both those conditions and other ones—for example, the rituals central to obsessive-compulsive disorders or the serious attention problems found in attention-deficit/hyperactivity disorder. Drugs, including low doses of medications such as Risperdal and Prozac, are also prescribed to reduce the aggressiveness and self-injury observed in some children with autism and the depression evident in some adolescents on the spectrum. Of course, all such drugs can have serious side effects and therefore should be administered with much caution, particularly with young children, and monitored carefully. (Both Risperdal and Prozac are currently being studied in NIH-supported research with children.) Some autistic children with epileptiform abnormalities on EEGs are being treated with Depakote.

The use of drugs with children has been severely criticized over the years. Consequently, many physicians have been reluctant to prescribe drug treatment for young children with autism, and many parents have rejected such treatment when it was offered. Indeed, in the hands of a physician not knowledgeable and experienced with this population, drug treatment can be harmful, particularly because dosages may be too high. Yet sometimes drug treatment can rescue a child and his or her family from the verge of disaster.

The behaviors that often lead to the use of drug treatment have been considered characteristics associated with autism. Recently, however, more attention has been given to the idea that such behaviors are comorbid neuropsychiatric disorders such as attention-deficit/hyperactivity disorder, obsessive-compulsive disorder, Tourette syndrome, and depression (Tsai 2001). Parents and individuals with autism, including Donna Williams, have suggested that what we call autism may reflect a combination of underlying conditions and that effective treatment may involve addressing each of these conditions.

Pharmacological treatment of autism has a long way to go. Fortunately, support for research into the biomedical factors in autism has increased dramatically since 1995, and many studies of drug treatment for children with autism are currently underway. The use of DNA as a variable in research on drug treatment has been proposed as a way of transforming pharmacology into a much more powerful treatment modality for autism in the future. Such research may enable us to dramatically refine and improve the system of prescribing medication.

Parents have played a major role in expanding research on autism. The National Alliance for Autism Research (NAAR) was formed in 1994 by a group of parents of children with autism. These parents were dismayed by the fact that autism research received much less funding from NIH than research on other conditions of similar or even lesser prevalence. The goal of NAAR was to advance biomedical research into the causes, prevention, treatment, and cure of autism spectrum disorders. Within a short period of time NAAR had designed several strategies for advancing autism research and began raising funds to implement this work. NAAR also collaborated with NIH and two other nongovernmental organizations in driving and shaping autism research for several years before merging with Autism Speaks in November 2005.

Cure Autism Now (CAN) is another group devoted to biomedical research and other routes to understanding and treating autism. It encourages and supports both basic research efforts and research that is closely linked to treatment. Founded in 1995 by the parents of a child with autism, this Los Angeles organization seeks to accelerate progress by funding cutting-edge research and by facilitating collaboration among researchers. It has made a major contribution by establishing a bank of genetics materials for researchers, and its advocacy efforts have played a significant part in securing more government funding. CAN is also collaborating with NIH on new autism research directions.

Research is taking us tantalizingly close to the answers we have been seeking about autism. Openness to the examination of all possibilities is the best route to ensuring that we do not overlook major factors involved in the behavior we identify by this label. The fact that one of the NIH-funded STAART centers is undertaking a major study of the role of gluten and casein in the functioning of children on the spectrum, despite the disdain and disparagement that many prominent professionals heaped on this possibility for years, is an encouraging development. While we define autism by its behavioral manifestations, in many children with autism multiple systems appear to have been affected, and multiple treatments may be the most effective means of helping these children overcome the imprisoning aspects of their condition. Moreover, the oft-repeated phrase "one size does not fit all" appears to be particularly appropriate in regard to individuals on the autism spectrum. We shouldn't be rejecting possibly useful hypotheses because they don't fit a majority of children on the spectrum. We need to take more seriously the possibility of small subgroups of children with autism spectrum disorders for whom particular treatments may be useful, although they may not serve any significant function for most other children on the spectrum.

In its 2001 report, *Educating Children with Autism,* the National Research Council, a major advisory group to the federal government, identified characteristics of effective educational interventions and made recommendations for improvement that are considered to represent best practice. Those characteristics included, for preschool children in particular, active engagement in a systematically planned instructional program for a minimum of twenty-five hours a week, twelve months a year, in a one-to-one format or in very small groups, with student-to-teacher ratios of not more than two to one. Other characteristics of effective educational programs are parent involvement, family support, use of highly trained staff, and ongoing assessment of child progress. An important question that can be asked is: How many young children with autism are in programs that meet these criteria?

Although we can't currently realize all our dreams for helping children with autism, we can do much more than we are doing today. We can, for example, work on the following strategies:

Use state-of-the-art techniques to identify infants and toddlers who may have an autism spectrum disorder. The infant/toddler section of IDEA, the federal education law focused on children with disabilities, calls for action aimed at early identification, but more strenuous efforts are needed, and they should reflect recent advances in early identification. Furthermore, such efforts should be targeted particularly at low-income families and other families with inexperienced, isolated, or overburdened parents. These are the families in which children with autism spectrum disorders are least likely to be identified early.

Provide intensive services to toddlers and preschoolers. The cost of intensive services for every toddler and preschooler diagnosed as having an autism spectrum disorder would undoubtedly be extremely high. But the current, sometimes feeble attempts at intervention for this population are unlikely to reduce the even greater costs of maintaining a large proportion of autistic individuals as seriously disabled throughout their lifetimes. It is cost-effective to help as many young children with autism as possible become part of the mainstream of society early in their lives, and we need intensive efforts to accomplish this. Not every toddler and preschooler who has an autism spectrum disorder will need twenty-five or more hours a week of educational intervention for an extended period; some children who begin receiving intensive services at age two or three will, not long after that, be able to learn effectively in small groups and benefit from supported participation in inclusive settings. But premature limitation of service time and premature reliance on group instruction are counterproductive strategies.

Redesign educational services for young school-age children, that is, children from five through seven, who have autism spectrum disorders. For those children who have not yet acquired speech, instruction should be heavily focused on establishing systems of communication. In the past, a significant number of autistic children—an estimated 50 percent—have not acquired functional speech. But among children who receive state-of-the-art intensive educational intervention starting at age two or three, that percentage is much lower, perhaps as small as 10 percent.

If a preschool child is not demonstrating progress in developing functional speech, an alternative mode of communication should be taught while speech instruction continues. This process requires blocks of one-to-one instructional time for students with teachers or speech/language therapists or both. A pre-kindergarten or kindergarten curriculum implemented primarily through group instruction does not constitute an adequate or appropriate instructional program for autistic children who lack functional language.

Instructional support is also needed in another vital area—namely, communicating, playing, and learning with typical children. A variety of strategies have been devised to develop such skills and to help children benefit from experiences in inclusive settings. At present, children with autism do not have sufficient opportunities for carefully planned, graduated, and adequately supported active participation in mainstream classes. Physical inclusion is a starting point, not an end point.

Make augmentative and alternative means of communication an integral part of the life of older students who do not have functional speech or whose speech is too limited to allow them to express their ideas fully. In one program for students with autism of high school age, I watched and listened to a small group discussion of a science topic being conducted in the school library. A boy of about sixteen did not participate, although he appeared to be alert to what was going on. I asked the program administrator about him and was told that although he was bright and could write, he couldn't speak. No pad, pen, pencil, typewriter, computer, or special communication device was in sight in the discussion area. Nor did the teacher request any communication from that student or address any questions or comments to him.

In addition to common tools for writing, a variety of special communication devices are available today for individuals of different ages and achievement levels. There is no excuse for any individual in any setting to be without an effective means of communication. We have been lax about ensuring that this does not occur; and we have not been vigorous enough in encouraging and supporting communication through an alternative mode when this is the only viable means of establishing functional communication. Professional passivity in this context fosters continued isolation and dependence for the autistic individual.

Provide more focused and intensive preparation for teachers in the strategies and skills needed to work productively with young children who have autism spectrum disorders. According to the report of the National Research Council: "Personnel preparation remains one of the weakest elements of effective programming for children with autistic spectrum disorders" (2001, 225).

While there are some commonalities in the learning needs of typical students or students with mild disabilities and students with autism, there are also many differences. It is not realistic to expect every teacher to have the skills needed to work with children who have autism, but it is reasonable to expect special education teachers to have such skills and to expect other teachers to receive in-service training, support, and supervision from professionals who have those skills. At the present time this is usually not what occurs.

In-service training is one mechanism for supplementing what teachers have learned in their college-based teacher education programs. It is a potentially valuable mechanism for developing better skills in the increasing number of teachers whose classes include students on the autism spectrum; and it is also essential to provide such training to their supervisors and school administrators. In-service training of college-level teacher educators is essential too. When parents began calling me in late 1993 seeking students to work in Lovaas-type in-home programs, I knew little about the most recent developments in the behavioral treatment of autistic children; and I was a teacher educator who had both experience and serious interest in the education of such children. What about the others?

Develop new strategies for matching educational intervention to the learning needs of individual children. During the last ten years or so, educational intervention has concentrated on refining, modifying, and merging elements of intervention methods. Although this process has been beneficial, we may now be approaching a point when a new direction is both warranted and possible. This path would be based on tools informed by advances in neuroimaging, genetics, and computer technology. It would be used to tie methodology more precisely to the learning modes and impediments of individual children, enabling parents and educators to identify intervention strategies that are more likely to be effective. Even the best intervention programs today only manage to help a portion of children with autism achieve close to normal functioning. There are still too many children we haven't been able to help enough.

We have been focusing on children with autism, but these children become adolescents and young adults with autism, and many of them continue to need special services or supports even if they do well in most areas of academic work. It would take another book to outline the kinds of educational assistance of benefit to older children, adolescents, and young adults. Without taking on this task, I will describe one aspect of such services. Educational planning for adolescents and young adults should revolve around the conceptualization of adult life for each particular individual. And how do we formulate this conceptualization? Fortunately, some very thoughtful professionals have been grappling with that question for well over a decade.

"Person-centered planning" is a term used to describe strategies to identify and pursue what a person with a disability wants and needs. The process starts by bringing together everyone who is significant in the person's life, including the individual himself or herself, with each participant sharing information about the individual's functioning and their vision for the person's future. The outcomes of this exploration are a picture of the overall themes that have an impact on the person's life and a vision of the future to be sought. Barriers to achieving that future and strategies for overcoming these barriers are also examined. This process differs from more common types of planning in several ways: it does not limit itself to one part of the person's life; the planning group is not limited to paid professionals and parents; and the current restrictions of service systems are not viewed as insurmountable obstacles that should narrow the options being considered for the life envisioned.

"Getting a life" is the overall theme and purpose of person-centered planning, and that's what happened to Jay Turnbull. Ann Turnbull, Jay's mother and a highly respected special educator, was a keynote speaker at the national conference of the Autism Society of America in 1995. The theme of her presentation was creating enviable lives for individuals with autism. Jay's family was unwilling to accept his life as it had become in young adulthood. And Jay communicated to them by his actions—head banging, hitting, choking, hair pulling, and refusal to get up in the morning—that his life was not the life that he wanted, either. The lifestyle that his family envisioned for him, and believed that Jay wanted too, was one of living, working, and participating in the community—not working in a large group of other people with severe disabilities at assembly-line packaging tasks, living with other people with severe disabilities, traveling in segregated groups, and interacting almost exclusively with other people with severe disabilities in a sheltered workshop or group home. Jay's family made a commitment to do everything necessary to help make Jay's envisioned life a reality.

The strategies the Turnbulls used to help Jay achieve a better life combined a person-centered planning process with positive behavioral supports. The planning process itself—the motivation, enthusiasm, and problem solving it generated—along with the intensive, comprehensive support system that developed during this process, enabled Jay, after a long and difficult period (which Ann Turnbull identified as about six years), to achieve the lifestyle envisioned for him. The criterion used to evaluate success was Jay's changed behavior: his greater independence, his part-time work, his enjoyment of music, his fun with family and friends, and the striking decrease in the challenging behaviors that he had exhibited. We do not yet know enough to enable most individuals with autism to attain enviable lives. Nor can most families put together the mixture of supports needed to attain such an outcome. But we have learned enough in recent years to help more and more individuals with autism go on to productive and satisfying lives.

We "typicals" carefully delineate the deficiencies of people with autism in being able to take the point of view of others, but can we ourselves switch lenses and look at the world from the perspective of people with autism? The Autism Network International (ANI) is a self-advocacy association of adults with autism spectrum disorders that evolved from a pen pal group facilitated by a parent organization. When a few of the members of this pen pal group met, they felt a sense of belonging, of being understood, of having the same concepts and sharing a language, of being "normal." Today the Autism Network International considers itself a community:

> In the last thirteen years, Autism Network International has grown from a small group of penpals meeting for the first time in a small apartment, to an international community of autistic people who meet online, in small informal meetings in private homes, and in our own communal space at Autreat. We have certain shared values in affirming the validity

of our way of being. We have many common experiences both with the experience of autism itself, and with being autistic in a world of neuro-typicals. . . . We have a dynamic, constantly-evolving set of customs and rules growing out of our shared experiences and our common needs. We have certain terms, expressions, and in-jokes that are distinct to our community. (Sinclair 2005)

A basic tenet of ANI is that "supports for autistic people should be aimed at helping them to compensate, navigate, and function in the world, not at changing them into non-autistic people or isolating them from the world" (Sinclair 2005). While many parents of young children with autism would not sign up for this philosophy—they want their children to be nonautistic—this position would be consistent with the goals of the parents of many older children, adolescents, and adults who continue to meet criteria for autism. In the 1990s ANI's newsletter was dominated by the themes of the struggle, discomfort, and distress of trying to relate to typical people; the battle to have pride in one's self as a person with autism; and the pleasure of relating to other people with autism. What these individuals found when they got together were friends with whom they could be themselves without being concerned about how their behavior looked in the world of typicals and without being asked to change.

Donna Williams was a contributor to the ANI newsletter, and one topic her contributions addressed was her attitude toward her own autism. The self-advocacy movement was strong among the members of this network, and some questioned Donna Williams's writings on this subject. She responded: "Autism is sometimes my sanctuary and sometimes my prison. When it imprisons me, I am at war with it. . . . The point is, not to fight autism per se, but to fight it *only for the right reasons*. . . . I will fight confinement wherever I find it" (Williams n.d., 6, 8).

There was much in those newsletters to make us question current conceptualizations of autism. True, the contributors represented only a tiny segment of the population of individuals with autism spectrum disorders, but they were not excluded from the generalizations about people with autism. Are people with autism unable to take the point of view of others, or do they have great difficulty with the process because the "others" in question are "typicals"? Do individuals with autism have this problem when the "others" are other people with autism? Are "typical" people any better at taking the viewpoint of people with autism than people with autism are in taking the point of view of "neurotypicals"? Researchers might do well to examine these questions.

Can people with autism have close friendships and adult love relationships? Many adults with autism have not had either, but that is not true of all people with autism, and it does not necessarily mean that they don't want such relationships. Some adolescents and adults on the spectrum very much want to have girlfriends or boyfriends and love relationships leading to marriage, and they actively pursue those possibilities. Temple Grandin concluded from her observations that "marriages work out best when two people with autism marry or when a person with autism marries . . . [an] eccentric spouse . . . [so that] their intellects work on a similar wavelength" (1995, 133). Sacks, in describing a married couple in which both people had Asperger syndrome, writes: "They recognized their own autism, and they had recognized each other's, at college, with a sense of such affinity and delight that it was inevitable they would marry. 'It was as if we had known each other for a million years,'" the wife remarked (1995, 276).

Yet some individuals with autism spectrum disorders do marry "typicals." Can such unions work? One mixed-marriage couple, writing in the ANI newsletter, reported that each of them had to work very hard at understanding the other, and each experienced culture shock. Yet what they also described was a close bond between them. The autistic husband felt very lucky to have found a partner like his wife, and the nonautistic wife reported that "for every time his autism drives me absolutely crazy, there are 4 or 5 times that it simply delights me" (Wiebe and Wiebe n.d., 15). Liane Willey writes of her relationship with her husband, who is her life support and partner:

> I know I would never have come this far if my husband had not been by my side. Not that our life together has always been easy. Like all married couples, we have had our share of problems, particularly when it comes to the one big issue that tears most marriages apart. The stuff of communicating.
>
> By the time I met my husband I was pretty well convinced I would

never understand anyone well enough to maintain something everlasting. The men I had been dating were nice men who shared some of my interests and hobbies, but with each of them there was always an unspoken and unseen something that stood between us. . . .

From the moment I met Tom, I sensed he was a great deal like me. . . . Like me, Tom dislikes crowds and social gatherings. He does not care for environments that are charged with emotion or chaos, and he does not care how he fits in with the rest of the world. Like me, he is a loner. (Willey 1999, 78–79)

Tom and Liane appear to mesh as a couple in spite of the fact that he is not on the spectrum. Does he have shadows of Asperger syndrome, or is his personality very close to that of a person with Asperger syndrome, like Liane? Whichever, that plus his openness and acceptance have allowed this relationship to flourish. Not so with other relationships in which "mixed couples" appear to love each other. Barbara Jacobs wrote a book entitled *Loving Mr. Spock,* which is almost an ode to her spectrum partner in a relationship that ultimately failed. "Believe me, loving an Asperger is not simple rocket science about women from Venus and men from Mars, but about loving a beautiful pretender from a parallel universe" (Jacobs 2003, 10). The gap between their universes proved too wide to be negotiated.

Putting aside for the moment the deficiencies and dysfunctions that occupy most of the attention of researchers and clinicians, we can cheer at some of the strengths of people with autism. One such strength is the continued learning throughout adulthood of some individuals with autism. Temple Grandin has grown greatly during her adult years—in self-awareness, in social skills, and in interpersonal relationships. She now talks about her friends and enjoys the company of those to whom she gives that designation. She has found ways of circumventing many of the imprisoning aspects of her autism, but she tells us, "I think lots of times there are things missing from my life." However, she also states, "if I could snap my fingers and be nonautistic, I would not—because then I wouldn't be me" (Sacks 1995, 286, 291). In November 2005, I marveled again at a painting by Jessy Park on exhibit at the Cooper Union in New

York City. This woman whose spoken words were still halting was able to create a vision of simple beauty from the prosaic experience of partially open doors showing a tree in a courtyard.

A mother of a boy with autism recounts:

> When I was fixing a snack in the kitchen for all my kids while they sat around the table doing homework, something about the situation reminded me of my mother, who'd died recently, and I began to quietly cry.
>
> My three younger children didn't notice. But my son looked up and said: What's wrong, Mom? Are you O.K.? and came over to give me a hug. I literally smiled through my tears.
>
> Somehow he had learned something they said couldn't be taught. I'll take that as a good sign. (LaZebnik 2005, 9)

Dreams live on. William and Barbara Christopher, parents of an adult son, had wishful dreams of their son being free of the confusion and pain that have marked much of his life. In these dreams Ned was married, had a good job, and made his own decisions. Those dreams did not come true for the Christophers, but we are approaching a point where the dreams of many other parents will.

APPENDIX A Diagnostic Criteria
for Autistic Disorder

A.   A total of six (or more) items from (1), (2), and (3), with at least two from (1), and one each from (2) and (3).

   (1)   qualitative impairment in social interaction, as manifested by at least two of the following:

      (a)   marked impairment in the use of multiple nonverbal behaviors such as eye-to-eye gaze, facial expression, body postures, and gestures to regulate social interaction

      (b)   failure to develop peer relationships appropriate to developmental level

      (c)   a lack of spontaneous seeking to share enjoyment, interests, or achievements with other people (e.g., by a lack of showing, bringing, or pointing out objects of interest)

      (d)   lack of social or emotional reciprocity

   (2)   qualitative impairments in communication as manifested by at least one of the following:

      (a)   delay in, or total lack of, the development of spoken language (not accompanied by an attempt to compensate through alternative modes of communication such as gesture or mime)

      (b)   in individuals with adequate speech, marked impairment in the ability to initiate or sustain a conversation with others

       (c)   stereotyped and repetitive use of language or idiosyncratic language

       (d)   lack of varied, spontaneous make-believe play or social imitative play appropriate to developmental level

  (3)   restricted repetitive and stereotyped patterns of behavior, interests, and activities, as manifested by at least one of the following:

       (a)   encompassing preoccupation with one or more stereotyped and restricted patterns of interest that is abnormal either in intensity or focus

       (b)   apparently inflexible adherence to specific, nonfunctional routines or rituals

       (c)   stereotyped and repetitive motor mannerisms (e.g., hand or finger flapping or twisting, or complex whole-body movements)

       (d)   persistent preoccupation with parts of objects

B.   Delays or abnormal functioning in at least one of the following areas, with onset prior to 3 years: (1) social interaction, (2) language as used in social communication, or (3) symbolic or imaginative play.

C.   The disturbance is not better accounted for by Rett's Disorder or Childhood Disintegrative Disorder.

APPENDIX B Diagnostic Criteria for Asperger's Disorder

A. Qualitative impairment in social interaction, as manifested by at least two of the following:
   (1) marked impairment in the use of multiple nonverbal behaviors such as eye-to-eye gaze, facial expression, body postures, and gestures to regulate social interaction
   (2) failure to develop peer relationships appropriate to developmental level
   (3) a lack of spontaneous seeking to share enjoyment, interests, or achievements with other people (e.g., by a lack of showing, bringing, or pointing out objects of interest to other people)
   (4) lack of social or emotional reciprocity
B. Restricted repetitive and stereotyped patterns of behavior, interests, and activities, as manifested by at least one of the following:
   (1) encompassing preoccupation with one or more stereotyped and restricted patterns of interest that is abnormal either in intensity or focus
   (2) apparently inflexible adherence to specific, nonfunctional routines or rituals

    (3)   stereotyped and repetitive motor mannerisms (e.g., hand or finger flapping or twisting, or complex whole-body movements)

    (4)   persistent preoccupation with parts of objects

C.   The disturbance causes clinically significant impairment in social, occupational, or other important areas of functioning.

D.   There is no clinically significant general delay in language (e.g., single words used by age 2 years, communicative phrases by 3 years).

E.   There is no clinically significant delay in cognitive development or in the development of age-appropriate self-help skills, adaptive behavior (other than social interaction), and curiosity about the environment in childhood.

F.   Criteria are not met for another specific Pervasive Developmental Disorder or Schizophrenia.

Resources

Please note that this list of resources is not meant to be exhaustive. It provides some major sources of information and assistance for parents and professionals who don't know how to proceed or want to learn more.

Autism Society of America
7910 Woodmont Avenue, Suite 300
Bethesda, Md. 20814–3067
Telephone: 800–3-AUTISM
Web site: www.autism-society.org

The Autism Society of America is a broad-based national organization that provides a variety of types of information services. It holds an annual national conference with a large number of presentations made to a diverse audience of family members, professionals, and individuals with autism spectrum disorders. There are multiple chapters of this organization across the country.

Autism Research Institute
4182 Adams Avenue
San Diego, Calif. 92116
Telephone: (619) 281–7165
Web site: www.autism.com/ari

The Autism Research Institute is a major resource for information on alternative treatment methods.

Autism Speaks
610 Fifth Avenue, Suite 604
New York, N.Y. 10020
Telephone: (212) 332–3580
Web site: www.autismspeaks.org

This organization merged with the National Alliance for Autism Research (NAAR) in late 2005. Its goal is to help find a cure for autism by raising funds to accelerate the pace of research and to raise public awareness. The web site contains information presented in visual and auditory formats.

Cure Autism Now (CAN) Foundation
5455 Wilshire Boulevard, Suite 2250
Los Angeles, Calif. 90036–4272
Telephone: (888) 828–8476
Web site: www.cureautismnow.org

This is an organization of parents, clinicians, and scientists dedicated to accelerating the pace of biomedical research. It raises funds for research projects on the causes, prevention, treatment, and cure for autism spectrum disorders. The web site provides basic information on autism as well as information on advocacy activities and research.

First Signs Inc.
P. O. Box 358
Merrimac, Mass. 01860
Telephone: (978) 346–4380
Web site: www.firstsigns.org

This organization is dedicated to early identification and treatment of autism spectrum disorders. It produces training materials for both families and professionals on "red flags."

Families for Early Autism Treatment (FEAT)
P. O. Box 255722
Sacramento, Calif. 95865–5722
Telephone (voicemail): (916) 463–5323
Web site: www.feat.org.

FEAT is a volunteer organization of parents and professionals dedicated to providing "world-class" education, advocacy, and support. It provides information, support, and assistance on evaluation and early intervention for parents of children with autism spectrum disorders.

Interdisciplinary Council on Developmental and Learning Disorders
4938 Hampden Lane, Suite 800
Bethesda, Md. 20814
Telephone: (301) 656–2667
Web site: www.icdl.com

This organization provides information and resources on the DIR/Floortime approach associated with Stanley Greenspan and Serena Wieder.

Lovaas Institute
(West Coast Headquarters)
11500 West Olympic Boulevard, Suite 318
Los Angeles, Calif. 90064
Telephone: (310) 914–5433
Web site: www.lovaas.com

The Lovaas Institute has multiple treatment centers across the country that offer clinic-based services to local families and consultation services to other families.

MAAP Services Inc.
P. O. Box 524
Crown Point, Ind. 46307
Telephone: (219) 662–1311
Web site: www.maapservices.org

MAAP Services for the Autism Spectrum is a nonprofit organization started by parents that provides information and advice to families of more advanced individuals with autism and Asperger syndrome.

Organization for Autism Research (OAR)
2111 Wilson Boulevard, Suite 600
Arlington, Va. 22201
Telephone: (703) 351–5031
Web site: www.researchautism.org

OAR's vision is to use science-based research to provide answers, practical alternatives, and solutions to the autism community. It supports applied research and offers free online guides to parents and professionals.

TEACCH
Treatment and Education of Autistic and Related Communication Handicapped Children
CB #7180
100 Renee Lynne Court
University of North Carolina at Chapel Hill
Chapel Hill, N.C. 27599–7180
Telephone: (919) 966–2174
Web site: www.teacch.com

TEACCH offers consultation and training to education and community agencies on various aspects of services to individuals with autism and their families, utilizing the approach developed by this system.

References

Abram, Samuel. 1999. *My corner.* Unpublished manuscript.

Adams, Christina. 2005. *A real boy: A true story of autism, early intervention, and recovery.* New York: Berkeley Books.

Advocate. 1994. Interview with Ivar Lovaas. *Advocate* 26 (November–December): 19–23.

———. 1995. An interview with Ruth Christ Sullivan. *Advocate* 27 (November–December): 9–15.

American Psychiatric Association. 2000. *Diagnostic and statistical manual of mental disorders.* 4th ed., Text Revision. Washington, D.C.: American Psychiatric Association.

Autism Research Institute. 2004. *Recovered autistic children.* DVD. Available from Autism Research Institute, 4182 Adams Avenue, San Diego, Calif., 92116.

———. 2005. *Autism is treatable! Science-based effective treatments. Proceedings of the Spring 2005 DAN! Conference.* Available from Autism Research Institute, 4182 Adams Avenue, San Diego, Calif., 92116.

Baron-Cohen, Simon, and Patricia Howlin. 1993. The theory of mind deficit in autism: Some questions for teaching and diagnosis. In *Understanding other minds: Perspectives from autism,* ed. Simon Baron-Cohen, Helen Tager-Flusberg, and Donald J. Cohen, 466–80. New York: Oxford University Press.

Barron, Judy, and Sean Barron. 1992. *There's a boy in here.* New York: Avon.

Bauman, Margaret L., and Thomas L. Kemper. 2005. Structural brain anatomy in autism: What is the evidence? In *The neurobiology of autism,* 2nd ed., ed. Margaret L. Bauman and Thomas L. Kemper, 121–35. Baltimore: Johns Hopkins University Press.

Bemporad, Jules R. 1979. Adult recollections of a formerly autistic child. *Journal of Autism and Developmental Disorders* 9: 179–97.

Biklen, Douglas. 1992. Autism orthodoxy versus free speech: A reply to Cummins and Prior. *Harvard Educational Review* 62: 242–56.

Billstedt, Eva, Carina Gillberg, and Christopher Gillberg. 2005. Autism after adolescence: Population-based 13- to 22-year follow-up study of 120 individuals with autism diagnosed in childhood. *Journal of Autism and Developmental Disorders* 35: 351–60.

Bondy, Andrew S., and Lori A. Frost. 1994. The Delaware autistic program. In *Preschool education programs for children with autism,* ed. Sandra L. Harris and Jan S. Handleman, 37–54. Austin, Tex.: PRO-ED.

Bovee, Jean-Paul. 1995. Jean-Paul. *Advocate* 27 (March-April): 6–7.

Brantlinger, Ellen A., Susan M. Klein, and Samuel L. Guskin. 1994. *Fighting for Darla: The case study of a pregnant adolescent with autism: Challenges for family care and professional responsibility.* New York: Teachers College Press.

Bruner, Jerome, and Carol Feldman. 1993. Theories of mind and the problem of autism. In *Understanding other minds: Perspectives from autism,* ed. Simon Baron-Cohen, Helen Tager-Flusberg, and Donald J. Cohen, 267–91. New York: Oxford University Press.

Bryson, Susan E. 2005. The autistic mind. In *The neurobiology of autism,* 2nd ed., ed. Margaret L. Bauman and Thomas L. Kemper, 34–44. Baltimore: Johns Hopkins University Press.

Callahan, Mary. 1987. *Fighting for Tony.* New York: Simon and Schuster.

Carpenter, Anne. 1992. Autistic adulthood: A challenging journey. In *High-functioning individuals with autism,* ed. Eric Schopler and Gary B. Mesibov, 289–94. New York: Plenum.

Carr, Edward G., Glen Dunlap, Robert H. Horner, Robert L. Koegel, Ann P. Turnbull, Wayne Sailor, Jacki L. Anderson, Richard W. Albin, Lynn K. Koegel, and Lise Fox. 2002. Positive behavior support: Evolution of an applied science. *Journal of Positive Behavior Interventions* 4: 4–16, 20.

Centers for Disease Control and Prevention. 2005. How common is Autism Spectrum Disorder (ASDs)? U.S. Department of Health and Human Services. Available online at www.cdc.gov/ncbddd/autism/asd_common.htm.

Cesaroni, Laura, and Malcolm Garber. 1991. Exploring the experience of autism through firsthand accounts. *Journal of Autism and Developmental Disorders* 21: 303–13.

Chakrabarti, Suniti, and Eric Fombonne. 2001. Pervasive developmental disorders in preschool children. *Journal of the American Medical Association* 285: 3093–99.

Chez, Michael. 2005. Improving core symptoms of language and social awareness in autism: Yes, medicine can help. Paper presented at the meeting of the Interdisciplinary Council on Developmental and Learning Disorders, McLean, Va., November.

Christopher, William, and Barbara Christopher. 1989. *Mixed blessings.* Nashville, Tenn.: Abingdon.

Church, Catherine C., and James Coplan. 1995. The high-functioning autistic experience: Birth to preteen years. *Journal of Pediatric Health Care* 9: 22–29.

Courchesne, Eric, Alan J. Lincoln, Jeanne P. Townsend, Hector E. James, Natacha A. Akshoomoff, Osamu Saitoh, Rachel Yeung-Courchesne, Brian Egaas, Gary A. Press, Richard H. Haas, James W. Murakami, and Laura Schreibman. 1994. A new finding: Impairment in shifting attention in autistic and cerebellar patients. In *Atypical cognitive deficits in developmental disorders: Implications for brain function,* ed. Sarah H. Broman and Jordan Grafman, 101–37. Hillsdale, N.J.: Lawrence Erlbaum.

Crimmins, Daniel, Anne F. Farrell, Philip W. Smith, and Alison Bailey. 2004. *Positive strategies: Developing individualized supports in schools.* Valhalla, N.Y.: Westchester Institute for Human Development.

Dawson, Geraldine. 1991. A psychobiological perspective on the early socioemotional development of children with autism. In *Rochester symposium on developmental psychopathology: Models and integrations,* ed. Dante Cicchetti and Sheree I. Toth, 3:207–34. Rochester, N.Y.: University of Rochester Press.

Dawson, Geraldine, Leslie J. Carver, Andrew N. Meltzoff, Heracles Panagiotides, James McPartland, and Sara J. Webb. 2002. Neural correlates of face and object recognition in young children with autism spectrum disorder, developmental delay, and typical development. *Child Development* 73: 700–717.

Dawson, Geraldine, and Renee Watling. 2000. Interventions to facilitate auditory, visual, and motor integration in autism: A review of the evidence. *Journal of Autism and Developmental Disorders* 30: 415–21.

DeMyer, Marian K., Sandra Barton, William E. DeMyer, James A. Norton, John Allen, and Robert Steele. 1973. Prognosis in autism: A follow-up study. *Journal of Autism and Childhood Schizophrenia* 3: 199–246.

DePaolo, Steffie. 1995. The ups and downs of silence. *Advocate* 27 (May–June): 9.

Dewey, Margaret. 1991. Living with Asperger's syndrome. In *Autism and Asperger syndrome,* ed. Uta Frith, 184–206. New York: Cambridge University Press.

Donnelly, Julia A. 1994. Excerpts from the young adults with autism panel: Speaking for ourselves, ASA 1994 Las Vegas. *Advocate* 26 (November–December): 7.

Donovan, William J. 1971. My experiences as an autistic child. In *Conference and* annual meeting of the National Society for Autistic Children, San Francisco, June 24–27, 1970, ed. Clara C. Park, 99–103. Public Health Services Publication no. 2164. Rockville, Md.: National Institute of Mental Health.

Eisenberg, Leon, and Leo Kanner. 1956. Childhood schizophrenia: Symposium, 1955–56. Early infantile autism, 1943–55. *American Journal of Orthopsychiatry* 26: 556–66.

Esch, Barbara E., and James E. Carr. 2004. Secretin as a treatment for autism: A review of the evidence. *Journal of Autism and Developmental Disorders* 34: 543–56.

Etscheidt, Susan. 2003. An analysis of legal hearings and cases related to individualized education programs for children with autism. *Research and Practice for Persons with Severe Disabilities* 28: 51–69.

Favell, Judith E. 2005. Sifting sound practice from snake oil. In *Controversial therapies for developmental disabilities: Fad, fashion, and science in professional practice*, ed. John W. Jacobson, Richard M. Foxx, and James A. Mulick, 19–30. Mahwah, N.J.: Lawrence Erlbaum.

Fein, Deborah, Pamela Dixon, Jennifer Paul, and Harriet Levin. 2005. Brief report: Pervasive Developmental Disorder can evolve into ADHD: Case illustrations. *Journal of Autism and Developmental Disorders* 35: 525–34.

Fling, Echo R. 2000. *Eating an artichoke: A mother's perspective on Asperger syndrome.* London: Jessica Kingsley Publishers.

Gajzago, Christine, and Margot Prior. 1974. Two cases of "recovery" in Kanner syndrome. *Archives of General Psychiatry* 31: 264–68.

Gardner, Howard. 1983. *Frames of mind: The theory of multiple intelligences.* New York: Basic Books.

———. 1993. *Multiple intelligences: The theory in practice.* New York: Basic Books.

Gernsbacher, Morton A. 2005. A parent's reflection. Paper presented at the meeting of the Interdisciplinary Council on Developmental and Learning Disorders, McLean, Va., November.

Gilbert, K. 1995. Preserving reality of autism. *Advocate* 27 (July–August): 4.

Gillberg, Christopher. 1991. Outcome in autism and autistic-like conditions. *Journal of the Academy of Child and Adolescent Psychiatry* 30: 375–82.

Gilpin, R. Wayne. 1993. *Laughing and loving with autism — a collection of "real life" warm and humorous stories.* Arlington, Tex.: Future Horizons.

———. 1994. *More laughing and loving with autism — a collection of "real life" warm and humorous stories.* Arlington, Tex.: Future Horizons.

Goodwin, Mary S., and T. Campbell Goodwin. 1969. In a dark mirror. *Mental Hygiene* 53: 550–63.

Grandin, Temple. 1995. *Thinking in pictures and other reports from my life with autism.* New York: Doubleday.

Grandin, Temple, and Catherine Johnson. 2005. *Animals in translation: Using the mysteries of autism to decode animal behavior.* New York: Scribner.

Grandin, Temple, and Margaret M. Scariano. 1986. *Emergence: Labeled autistic.* Novato, Calif.: Arena.

Gray, Carol A. 1995. Teaching children with autism to "read" social situations. In *Teaching children with autism: Strategies to enhance communication and socialization,* ed. Kathleen Ann Quill, 219–41. New York: Delmar.

Greenfeld, Josh. 1972. *A child called Noah: A family journey.* New York: Holt, Rinehart and Winston.

———. 1978. *A place for Noah.* New York: Harcourt Brace Jovanovich.

Greenspan, Stanley I., and Serena Wieder. 1998. *The child with special needs: Encouraging intellectual and emotional growth.* Reading, Mass.: Addison-Wesley.

———. 1999. A functional developmental approach to autism spectrum disorders. *Journal of the Association for Persons with Severe Handicaps* 24: 147–61.

———. 2005. The ICDL Diagnostic Manual. Paper presented at the meeting of the Interdisciplinary Council on Developmental and Learning Disorders, McLean, Va., November.

Gutstein, Steven E. 2000. *Autism Aspergers: Solving the relationship puzzle.* Arlington, Tex,: Future Horizons.

Hall, Kenneth. 2001. *Asperger syndrome, the universe and everything.* London: Jessica Kingsley Publishers.

Hamilton, Lynn M. 2000. *Facing autism: Giving parents reasons for hope and guidance for help.* Colorado Springs: Waterbrook.

Happe, Francesca. 1991. The autobiographical writings of three Asperger syndrome adults: Problems of interpretation and implications for theory. In *Autism and Asperger syndrome,* ed. Uta Frith, 207–42. New York: Cambridge University Press.

Harland, Kelly. 2002. *A will of his own: Reflections on parenting a child with autism.* Bethesda, Md.: Woodbine House.

Harris, Sandra L. 1994. *Siblings of children with autism: A guide for families.* Bethesda, Md.: Woodbine House.

———. 2005. Ask the editor. *Journal of Autism and Developmental Disorders* 35: 137.

Hart, Charles. 1989. *Without reason: A family copes with two generations of autism.* New York: Harper and Row.

Hazlett, Heather C., Michele Poe, Guido Gerig, Rachel G. Smith, James Provenzale, Allison Ross, John Gilmore, and Joseph Piven. 2005. Magnetic resonance imaging and head circumference study of brain size in autism: Birth through age 2 years. *Archives of General Psychiatry* 62: 1366–76.

Howard, Jane S., Coleen R. Sparkman, Howard G. Cohen, Gina Green, and Harold Stanislaw. 2005. A comparison of intensive behavior analytic and eclectic treatments for young children with autism. *Research in Developmental Disabilities* 26: 359–83.

Hundley, Joan M. 1971. *The small outsider: The story of an autistic child.* New York: St. Martin's Press.

Hurlburt, Russell T., Francesca Happe, and Uta Frith. 1994. Sampling the form of inner experience in three adults with Asperger syndrome. *Psychological Medicine* 24: 385–95.

Isaiah. 1995. A brother's view. *Advocate* 27 (September–October): 7.

Jacobs, Barbara. 2003. *Loving Mr. Spock: Understanding an aloof lover.* Arlington, Tex.: Future Horizons.

Jacobson, John W., Richard M. Foxx, and James A. Mulick. 2005. Facilitated communication: The ultimate fad. In *Controversial therapies for developmental disabilities: Fad, fashion, and science in professional practice,* ed. John W. Jacobson, Richard M. Foxx, and James A. Mulick, 363–83. Mahwah, N.J.: Lawrence Erlbaum.

Johnson, Carol, and Julia Crowder. 1994. *Autism: From tragedy to triumph.* Boston: Brandon Books.

Kanner, Leo. 1973. *Childhood psychosis: Initial studies and new insights.* Washington, D.C.: Winston.

Kaufman, Barry N. 1976. *Son rise.* New York: Warner Books.

———. 1994. *Son rise: The miracle continues.* Tiburon, Calif.: Kramer.

Kennedy, Diane. 2002. *The ADHD autism connection: A step toward more accurate diagnosis and effective treatment.* Colorado Springs: Waterbrook Press.

Kiebala, Eileen S. 1995. Patrick. *Advocate* 27 (July–August): 10–11.

Kirby, David. 2005. *Evidence of harm: Mercury in vaccines and the autism epidemic: A medical controversy.* New York: St. Martin's Press.

Koegel, Lynn K., and Claire LaZebnik. 2004. *Overcoming autism: Finding the answers, strategies, and hope that can transform a child's life.* New York: Viking.

Koegel, Robert L., and Lynn K. Koegel. 2005. *Pivotal response treatments for autism: Communication, social, and academic development.* Baltimore: Paul H. Brookes.

Koplow, Lesley, Suzanne Abrams, Judy Ferber, and Beverly Dennis. 1996. Helping children with pervasive developmental disorders. In *Unsmiling faces: How preschools can heal,* ed. Lesley Koplow, 181–201. New York: Teachers College Press.

LaZebnik, Claire. 2005. Adolescence, without a roadmap. *New York Times,* October 16, Sunday Styles, 9.

Leakey, Richard. 1994. *The origin of humankind.* New York: Basic Books.

Lord, Catherine, and Eric Schopler. 1989a. The role of age at assessment, developmental level, and test in the stability of intelligence scores in young autistic children. *Journal of Autism and Developmental Disorders* 19: 483–99.

———. 1989b. Stability of assessment results of autistic and non-autistic language-impaired children from preschool years to early school age. *Journal of Child Psychology and Psychiatry* 30: 575–90.

Lord, Catherine, Michael Rutter, and Ann Le Couteur. 1994. Autism Diagnostic Interview–Revised: A revised version of a diagnostic interview for caregivers of individuals with possible pervasive developmental disorders. *Journal of Autism and Developmental Disorders* 24: 659–85.

Lord, Catherine, Michael Rutter, Pamela C. DiLavore, and Susan Risi. 2002. *Autism Diagnostic Observation Schedule.* Los Angeles, Calif.: Western Psychological Services.

Lotter, Victor. 1978. Follow-up studies. In *Autism: A reappraisal of concepts and treatment,* ed. Michael Rutter and Eric Schopler, 475–95. New York: Plenum.

Lovaas, O. Ivar. 1987. Behavioral treatment and normal educational and intellectual functioning in young autistic children. *Journal of Consulting and Clinical Psychology* 55: 3–9.

———.2003. *Teaching individuals with developmental delays: Basic intervention techniques.* Austin, Tex.: PRO-ED.

Lovaas, O. Ivar, and Gregory Buch. 1997. Intensive behavioral intervention with young children with autism. In *Prevention and treatment of severe behavior problems: Models and method in developmental disabilities,* ed. Nirbhay N. Singh, 61–86. Pacific Grove, Calif.: Brooks/Cole.

Makarushka, M. 1991. The words they can't say. *New York Times Magazine,* October 6, 32–33, 36, 70.

Marks, Susan U., Carl Schrader, Trish Longaker, and Mark Levine. 2000. Portraits of three adolescent students with Asperger's syndrome: Personal stories and how they can inform practice. *Journal of the Association for Persons with Severe Handicaps* 25: 3–17.

Maurice, Catherine. 1993. *Let me hear your voice: A family's triumph over autism.* New York: Fawcett Columbine.

Maurice, Catherine, Gina Green, and Stephen C. Luce, eds. 1996. *Behavioral intervention for young children with autism: A manual for parents and professionals.* Austin, Tex.: PRO-ED.

McDonnell, Jane T. 1993. *News from the border: A mother's memoir of her autistic son.* New York: Ticknor and Fields.

McEachin, John J., Tristram Smith, and O. Ivar Lovaas. 1993. Long-term outcome for children with autism who received early intensive behavioral treatment. *American Journal on Mental Retardation* 97: 359–72.

McKean, Thomas A. 1994. *Soon will come the light: A view from inside the autism puzzle.* Arlington, Tex.: Future Education.

Mesibov, Gary B., Victoria Shea, and Eric Schopler. 2004. *The TEACCH approach to autism spectrum disorders.* New York: Springer.

Miller, Arnold, and Ellen Eller-Miller. 1989. *From ritual to repertoire: A cognitive-developmental systems approach with behavior-disordered children.* New York: Wiley.

Mirenda, Patricia L., and Anne M. Donnellan. 1987. Issues in curriculum development. In *Handbook of autism and pervasive developmental disorders,* ed. Donald J. Cohen, Anne M. Donnellan, and Rhea Paul, 211–26. New York: Wiley.

Morphett, Lurline. 1986. *Face to face.* South Australia: Education Department of South Australia.

National Institute of Mental Health. 2005. NIH joined by advocacy groups to fund research on autism susceptibility genes. Press release. October 18. Available online at www.nimh.nih.gov/press/autismconsortiumgrants.cfm.

National Research Council. 2001. *Educating children with autism.* Committee on Educational Interventions for Children with Autism. Ed. Catherine Lord and James. P. McGee, Division of Behavioral and Social Sciences and Education. Washington, D.C.: National Academy Press.

Nickelsen, Fallon. 1996. Erik. *Advocate* 28 (March–April): 4.

Pangborn, Jon, and Sidney M. Baker. 2005. *Autism: Effective biomedical treatments.* San Diego, Calif.: Autism Research Institute.

Paradiz, Valerie. 2002. *Elijah's cup: A family's journey into the community and culture of high-functioning autism and Asperger's syndrome.* New York: Free Press.

Park, Clara Claiborne. 1982. *The siege: The first eight years of an autistic child, with an epilogue, fifteen years later.* Boston: Little, Brown.

———. 1986. Social growth in autism: A parent's perspective. In *Social behavior in autism,* ed. Eric Schopler and Gary B. Mesibov, 81–99. New York: Plenum.

———, ed. 1971. *Conference and annual meeting of the National Society for Autistic Children, San Francisco, June 24–27, 1970.* Public Health Services Publication no. 2164. Rockville, Md.: National Institute of Mental Health.

Pinney, Rachel, and Mimi Schlachter. 1983. *Bobby: Breakthrough of a special child.* New York: St. Martin's Press/Marek.

Prizant, Barry M., and Amy M. Wetherby. 1989. Providing services to children with autism ages 0–2 and their families. *Focus on Autistic Behavior* 4 (2): 1–16.

Rapoport, Judith L. 1989. *The boy who couldn't stop washing: The experience and treatment of obsessive-compulsive disorder.* New York: New American Library.

Ratey, John J., and Catherine Johnson. 1997. *Shadow syndromes.* New York: Pantheon Books.

Rimland, Bernard. 1964. *Infantile autism: The syndrome, and its implications for a neural theory of behavior.* New York: Appleton-Century-Crofts.

Robins, Diana L., Deborah Fein, Marianne L. Barton, and James A. Green. 2001. The Modified Checklist for Autism in Toddlers: An initial study investigating the early detection of autism and pervasive developmental disorders. *Journal of Autism and Developmental Disorders* 31: 131–44.

Rutter, Michael. 1983. Cognitive deficits in the pathogenesis of autism. *Journal of Child Psychology and Psychiatry* 24: 513–31.

Sacks, Oliver. 1995. *An anthropologist on Mars: Seven paradoxical tales.* New York: Knopf.

Sallows, Glen O., and Tamlynn D. Graupner. 2005. Intensive behavioral treatment for children with autism: Four-year outcome and predictors. *American Journal on Mental Retardation* 110: 417–38.

Schulte-Hillen, K. H. 1969. My search to find the drug that crippled my baby. In *If your child is handicapped*, ed. William C. Kvaraceus and E. Nelson Hayes, 37–52. Boston: Porter Sargent.

Schulze, Craig B. 1993. *When snow turns to rain: One family's struggle to solve the riddle of autism*. Rockville, Md.: Woodbine House.

Seroussi, Karyn. 2000. *Unraveling the mystery of autism and pervasive developmental disorder: A mother's story of research and recovery*. New York: Simon and Schuster.

Serra, Marike, M. Althaus, L. M. J. de Sonneville, A. D. Stant, A. E. Jackson, and R. B. Minderaa. 2003. Face recognition in children with a pervasive developmental disorder not otherwise specified. *Journal of Autism and Developmental Disorders* 33: 303–17.

Shore, Stephen. 2003. *Beyond the wall: Personal experiences with autism and Asperger syndrome*. 2nd ed. Shawnee Mission, Kans.: Autism Asperger Publishing.

Sinclair, J. 1992. Bridging the gaps: An inside-out view of autism. In *High-functioning individuals with autism*, ed. Eric Schopler and Gary B. Mesibov, 294–302. New York: Plenum.

———. 2005. Autism Network International: The development of a community and its culture. January. Available online at http://web.syr.edu/~jisincla/History_of_ANI.html.

Smith, Tristram, and Michelle Antolovich. 2000. Parental perceptions of supplemental interventions received by young children with autism in intensive behavior analytic treatments. *Behavioral Interventions* 15: 83–97.

Smith, Tristram, Svein Eikeseth, Morten Klevstrand, and O. Ivar Lovaas. 1997. Intensive behavioral treatment for preschoolers with severe mental retardation and pervasive developmental disorder. *American Journal on Mental Retardation* 102: 238–49.

Smith, Tristram, Daniel W. Mruzek, and Dennis Mozingo. 2005. Sensory integration therapy. In *Controversial therapies for developmental disabilities: Fad, fashion, and science in professional practice*, ed. John W. Jacobson, Richard M. Foxx, and James A. Mulick, 331–50. Mahwah, N.J.: Lawrence Erlbaum.

Stehli, Annabel. 1991. *The sound of a miracle*. New York: Avon Books.

Steingard, Ronald J., Daniel F. Connor, and Trang Au. 2005. Approaches to psychopharmacology. In *The neurobiology of autism*, 2nd ed., ed. Margaret L. Bauman and Thomas L. Kemper, 79–102. Baltimore: Johns Hopkins University Press.

Strain, Phillip S., and Marilyn Hoyson. 2000. The need for longitudinal, intensive social skill intervention: LEAP follow-up outcomes for children with autism. *Topics in Early Childhood Special Education* 20: 116–22.

Strain, Phillip S., Frank W. Kohler, and Howard Goldstein. 1996. Learning experiences . . . an alternative program: Peer mediated interventions for young children with autism. In *Child and adolescent disorders: Empirically based strate-*

gies for clinical practice, ed. Euthymia D. Hibbs and Peter S. Jensen, 573–87. Washington, D.C.: American Psychological Association.

Sundberg, Mark L., and James W. Partington. 1998. *Teaching language to children with autism or other developmental disabilities.* Pleasant Hills, Calif.: Behavior Analysts.

Szatmari, Peter, Giampierro Bartolucci, R. Bremner, S. Bond, and S. Rich. 1989. A follow-up study of high-functioning autistic children. *Journal of Autism and Developmental Disorders* 19: 213–25.

Taylor, Bridget A., and Kelly A. McDonough. 1996. Selecting teaching programs. In *Behavioral intervention for young children with autism,* ed. Catherine Maurice, Gina Green, and Stephen C. Luce, 63–177. Austin, Tex.: PRO-ED.

Tsai, Luke. 2001. *Taking the mystery out of medications in autism/Asperger syndromes: A guide for parents and non-medical professionals.* Arlington, Tex.: Future Horizons.

U.S. Government Accountability Office. 2005. *Special education: Children with autism.* GAO-05–220. Washington, D.C.: U.S. Government Accountability Office.

Volkmar, Fred R. 1993. Autism and the pervasive developmental disorders. In *Handbook of infant mental health,* ed. Charles H. Zeanah, 236–49. New York: Guilford.

Volkmar, Fred R., and Donald J. Cohen. 1985. The experience of infantile autism: A first-person account by Tony W. *Journal of Autism and Developmental Disorders* 15: 47–54.

Volkmar, Fred R., and Lisa A. Wiesner. 2004. *Healthcare for children on the autism spectrum: A guide to medical, nutritional, and behavioral issues.* Bethesda, Md.: Woodbine House.

Warren, Frank. 1984. The role of the national society in working with families. In *The effects of autism on the family,* ed. Eric Schopler and Gary B. Mesibov, 99–115. New York: Plenum.

Werner, Emily, and Geraldine Dawson. 2005. Validation of the phenomenon of autistic regression using home videotapes. *Archives of General Psychiatry* 62: 889–95.

White, B. B., and M. S. White. 1987. Autism from the inside. *Medical Hypotheses* 24: 223–29.

Wiebe, Lauren, and Dan Wiebe. n.d. She says, he says: Progress reports from a mixed marriage. *Our Voice* 1 (4): 15–16.

Willey, Liane H. 1999. *Pretending to be normal.* London: Jessica Kingsley Publishers.

———. 2002. *Asperger syndrome in the family: Redefining normal.* London: Jessica Kingsley Publishers.

Williams, Donna. 1992. *Nobody nowhere: The extraordinary autobiography of an autistic.* New York: Times Books.

———. 1994a. Invited commentary: In the real world. *Journal of the Association for Persons with Severe Handicaps* 19: 196–99.

————. 1994b. *Somebody somewhere: Breaking free from the world of autism.* New York: Times Books.

————. 1996. *Autism — an inside-out approach: An innovative look at the mechanics of "autism" and its developmental "cousins."* London: Jessica Kingsley Publishers.

————. n.d. About "fighting autism." *Our Voice* 2 (1): 6–8.

Williams, Justin H. G., Andrew Whiten, and Tulika Singh. 2004. A systematic review of action imitation in autistic spectrum disorder. *Journal of Autism and Developmental Disorders* 34: 285–99.

Zatlow, Gerri. 1982. A sister's lament. *Exceptional Parent* 12: 50–51.

ADDITIONAL READINGS

Bashe, Patricia R. and Barbara L. Kirby. 2005. *The OASIS guide to Asperger syndrome: Advice, support, insight, and inspiration.* Rev. ed. New York: Crown.

Cohen, Shirley. 2006. Inclusion of young children with autism spectrum disorders: Updates and other thoughts. *Autism Asperger's Digest Magazine* (May-June). In press.

Exkorn, Karen S. 2005. *The autism sourcebook: Everything you need to know about diagnosis, treatment, coping, and healing.* New York: Regan Books.

Gutstein, Steven E., and Rachelle K. Sheely. 2002. *Relationship development intervention with young children: Social and emotional development activities for Asperger syndrome, autism, PDD, and NLD.* London: Jessica Kingsley Publishers.

Handleman, Jan S., and Sandra Harris, eds. 2001. *Preschool education programs for children with autism.* 2nd ed. Austin, Tex.: PRO-ED.

New York State Department of Health, Early Intervention Program. 1999. *Clinical practice guideline: Report of the recommendations, autism/pervasive developmental disorders, assessment and intervention for young children (age 0–3 years).* Publication no. 4215. Albany, N.Y.

Shea, Victoria. 2004. A perspective on the research literature related to early intensive behavioral intervention (Lovaas) for young children with autism. *Autism* 8: 349–67.

Wetherby, Amy M., and Barry M. Prizant, eds. 2000. *Autism spectrum disorders: A transactional developmental perspective.* Baltimore: Paul Brookes.

Wiseman, Nancy D. 2006. *Could it be autism? A parent's guide to the first signs and next steps.* New York: Broadway Books.

Zero to Three/National Center for Clinical Infant Programs. 2005. DC: 0–3R: *Diagnostic classification of mental health and developmental disorders of infancy and early childhood.* Rev. ed. Arlington, Va.: National Center for Clinical Infant Programs.

Index

ABA. *See* applied behavior analysis
ABC *Day One*, 18
abuse: by family members, 82–83, 171; of individuals with disabilities, 171. *See also* self-injurious behavior
accommodation: adaptation combined with, 80, 129–30; FC and, 170; TEACCH, 126, 128–30
acquired epileptic aphasia, 19. *See also* Landau-Kleffner syndrome
Adams, Christina: combining intervention treatments, 131–32; *A Real Boy* on parent categories, 153–54; on recovery, 191
Adams, Jonah: combined treatments, 131–32; medication, 162; and recovery, 191; tantrums, 61
ADHD (attention-deficit/hyperactivity disorder), 7, 21–22, 66, 159, 191, 197
The ADHD-Autism Connection (Kennedy), 22
adolescence, 68–77, 119, 201, 202–3
adulthood, 41, 203–7; continued learning throughout, 207; marriages, 178, 189, 206–

7; networks, 190, 204–5; planning for, 73, 203–4; self-advocacy movement, 30, 38–40, 204–5; sensory hypersensitivity, 32; young, 68–77, 202–3. *See also* parents
Advocate, 83, 89, 141
African American woman, at Westchester conference, 94, 99–100, 147–48
aggression: ABA treatment and, 131; adolescence and young adulthood, 69, 75–76; medications, 61, 197; in meltdowns, 61; middle childhood, 59, 61, 101; parental stress and, 85, 101
AIT (auditory integration training), 81, 164–65
alienness: insider descriptions, 36–38. *See also* differentness
American Academy of Neurology, 106
American Academy of Pediatrics, 106
American Psychiatric Association (APA), 4–5
American Psychologist, 168
amygdala, 195

Text: 10/14 Palatino
Display: Bauer Bodoni and Univers Condensed
Compositor: BookMatters, Berkeley
Printer and binder: Maple-Vail Manufacturing Group